THE Y PLAN

First published in Great Britain in 1990

This edition published in 1995 by Virgin Books,
an imprint of Virgin Publishing Ltd
332 Ladbroke Grove, London W10 5AH

The Stress Care questionnaire on page 131 is reproduced courtesy of Stress Care,
7 Park Crescent, London W1N 3HE. Tel: 0181–594 4488

A catalogue record for this book is available from the British Library

ISBN: 086369 981 2

Designed by Graham Davis Associates
Photographs by Peter Mason
Additional illustrations by Alex Ayliffe
Cover design by Slatter-Anderson

Typeset by Phoenix Photosetting, Chatham, Kent
Printed and bound in Great Britain by
Butler & Tanner Ltd, Frome and London

THE Y PLAN

THE 12 MINUTE WAY TO *TOTAL* *FITNESS*

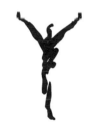

WITH

ANTHEA TURNER

We owe grateful thanks to Dr Craig Sharp and Leo Foulman of the British Olympic Medical Centre for their help, advice and encouragement, and in particular to Craig Sharp for his comments and criticisms on the text of this book.

We would also like to make acknowledgement to: Rodney Cullum, Operations Director at London Central YMCA; Gemma Raimondo and Scotti Macdonald for being such willing guinea-pigs in Craig Sharp's fitness test class; Pamela Etheridge, Robin Gargrave, Tony Odinoye and, of course, Anthea Turner for undertaking all the exercises photographed for this book; Lucy Wagner at Virgin Lifetime Video for her assistance; and the entire staff of London Central YMCA Training and Development Department for their unfailing support.

Dr Craig Sharp is Director of the British Olympic Medical Centre in Middlesex and was formerly co-director of the British Human Motor Performance Laboratory at the University of Birmingham. He is one of Britain's leading physiologists.

Anthea Turner began her career in local radio in Staffordshire but since 1986 has concentrated more on television and video presentation. She has a background of training in ballet at the Royal Academy of Dance and holds a teaching certificate in tap dancing.

Lesley Mowbray, Director, Training and Development, YMCA, is the leading figure in Britain for fitness teacher-training. She graduated in Art and Science of Movement from Dartford College in Kent and is the co-author of two books, *English YMCA Guide to Exercise to Music* and *The Teaching of Health-Related Exercise*, based on courses she has developed. She has also acted as consultant on two Virgin Lifetime videos, *Sensible Slimming* and *Body Maintenance*. She lectures, directs workshops and seminars on exercise to music, including a course on *Teaching the Fifty-Plus*, and is increasingly involved in researching and developing other new courses, all of which are RSA/Sport Council-approved, to safeguard standards of safety and effectiveness.

Jill Gaskell, Deputy Director, Training and Development, YMCA, graduated in Sport, Science and Physical Education from Loughborough University and has also studied fitness in New Zealand. With Lesley Mowbray, she was instrumental in setting up a course for Ante/Post-Natal Exercise. She has appeared on television, radio and video, and has run courses and workshops on fitness throughout Britain.

CONTENTS

Preface

There is excellent evidence that exercise is beneficial to physical health. Professors Jerry Morris in London, and Ralph Paffenbargar in the USA, pioneered studies which demonstrated a lowered incidence of coronary heart disease and related disorders in subjects who took regular exercise. Recently, Dr Adrianno Hardman at Loughborough has shown in women subjects that the level of exercise required to cause health benefits does not need to be excessively hard. Indeed, her study was done on walking.

More and more evidence is accumulating to suggest that modest exercise programmes may benefit psychological health as well as physical. For example, Professor Hannah Steinberg in London believes that even mild physical activity, on a regular basis, can alleviate symptoms of stress and depression. She is an advocate simply of a more active lifestyle involving housework, walking and gardening, all performed more vigorously than before.

Apart from health and psychological well-being, being fitter in terms of heart and muscle and flexible joints can make many aspects of day-to-day living easier, including carrying the shopping, going up hills or long flights of stairs, playing with one's vigorous children, hurrying for buses, trains or appointments – right down to such simple tasks as cutting one's toe nails or tying one's shoe laces; all are correspondingly easier, the fitter and more flexible one is.

That is the brief case for exercise, but *how* to exercise is a problem for many. There are numerous books and video tapes on exercise and many have their good points, although equally many contain unsafe exercise elements and are written or produced by authors who have little or no underlying knowledge of exercise science or physiology.

The authors of the Y Plan have spent several years getting it right. They are a pair of very able young women, well trained in exercise and enormously experienced in training exercise teachers and in running exercise programmes at the famous Central London YMCA Fitness and Health Centre. From time to time I have met one or both of them at scientific conferences on various aspects of exercise, and I have always been impressed by their determination to enlarge their knowledge on the scientific side and to keep up to date.

Exercise is undeniably very good for you and the Y Plan is a very good graded exercise programme into which a lot of thought has gone as to its effectiveness and safety. I have a friend, Jackie Dickinson, who is no doubt typical of tens of thousands of working wives with children who wish and indeed need to exercise, but who needs a structured format in which she can have confidence.

For her and all like her – and their male counterparts – all with very limited time to spare, the Y Plan is absolutely ideal. It is short, effective, safe and scientifically as sound as the state of current knowledge. This is a very 'user-friendly' exercise programme, which is just as well, because in order to gain life-long benefits from exercise, you have to exercise consistently for the rest of your life.

Dr N C Craig Sharp BVMS, MRCVS, PhD, FIBiol
Director
British Olympic Medical Centre

Introduction

....

Welcome to the Y Plan.

Most people can be convinced that there is a *need* for exercise. After all, we are not the only people promoting the value of it – magazines, newspapers, television and doctors bombard everyone with similar information. The real challenge is to motivate people from the stage of understanding the need for exercise to actually starting and sticking to a regular exercise plan.

Neither trendy gimmicks nor the latest 'incredible' fad is the answer. Too often people who are prepared to have a go find what they are asked to do too difficult or time-consuming or they find that the latest hype is not all it claims to be, and consequently they get discouraged and probably give up. Some fitness plans go to the other extreme in persuading people to go for one simple idea: their exercises involve holding a position for a certain time, and that will do the trick. This type of static exercise is known as isometric and people need to be aware that it can lead to a rapid rise in blood pressure, which could be very dangerous. In any case, its effects in improving overall fitness are limited. As safety and effectiveness are our priorities, the Y Plan avoids all isometric and specific static exercise.

The Y Plan is based on fitness facts and an in-depth understanding of body function and mechanics. It combines two types of exercise. Muscular toning, which works individual muscles and creates a firm, shapely body, and aerobic exercise, which works the large muscle groups – the heart, the lungs and the circulatory system. These exercises improve the body's energy-capability and its co-ordination (known as motor fitness) at the same time as improving body shape.

Instead of having to set aside long periods of time to go through a home exercise class, the Y Plan only needs twelve minutes of your time for exercise, every other day, and in as little as five weeks you will be able to see and feel the difference in yourself. It has three ascending levels, through which you progress as fast and as far as you can. You will be given clear guidelines to establish the right starting level for you so that you can be completely confident that you are taking part in an exercise programme that exactly suits your own capacities and needs. Once you are under way with the programme you will soon find both that exercise is enjoyable and that it gives you a great sense of achievement. More than that, the Y Plan will make you look great and feel terrific.

If you have any doubt about whether or not you should exercise, however, don't hesitate to seek the advice of your local doctor.

The Y Plan is scientifically based so that it is effective and safe. The London Central YMCA is part of a worldwide organisation whose aims are to meet the needs of its community. The YMCA organisation of the USA has for many years taken the leading role in educating Americans in health and fitness issues through numerous books and national fitness programmes. In Britain, Rodney Cullum, the London Central YMCA's Physical Education Director, developed a fresh philosophy and direction for its physical education programme, with training programmes that have been devised in co-operation with the sports science faculty at Loughborough University.

Our major task in the last twelve years has been to convince all kinds of men and women of the need to exercise. We have talked to them; quoted statistics from doctors and experts at them; and, most of all, provided carefully constructed and varied exercise programmes to fit their individual needs. Up and down Britain there are literally thousands of classes, either in YMCAs or in other fitness studios, being led by LCYMCA/Royal Society of Arts/Sports Council-trained teachers, and any of these instructors will be able to help you get the best out of your Y Plan programme. It's that easy – call in to see when there's a class that suits your arrangements and you'll be on your way to getting fitter, looking better and probably to making new friends in the process. Somewhere in your area, the Y Plan is at work!

Our experience has taught us many things, one of which is that all types of people of all ages can be persuaded to take up regular exercise. Their motives and even their

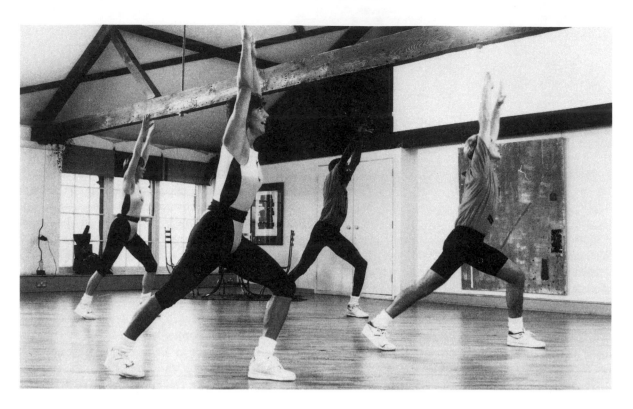

rewards may differ widely, but all will benefit.

When we are young, fitness and shape should come naturally. Our muscles are firm and strong, our hearts are lively and healthy, and our limbs are nimble and flexible. Our self-image is good and our attitude to all around us is simple and direct. We have usually not experienced either the physical or mental wear and tear of life. As we grow older we actively avoid strenuous activity, driving instead of walking, using lifts and escalators rather than stairs. We may kid ourselves that it's to save time but however it is, our lives become increasingly inactive, both in our work and leisure activities.

The Y fitness classes have become a haven for people who have recognised this attitude in themselves. From clerks to cabbies, mothers to models, bankers to bakers, vicars to viscounts, secretaries to starlets, the Y classes have helped to boost confidence, enhance self-image and body shape, and improve all-round health and fitness.

Because exercise is a long-term investment in staying in shape and keeping fat at bay, too many people are tempted instead by the latest, quick diets. Research suggests that only 5–10 per cent of dieters successfully maintain any weight loss they achieve by this means. At Y classes we come across hundreds of people who have failed to control their body weight. Among many different age groups the pattern tends to be the same. The weight gain has been

very gradual – an average fairly sedentary person tends to gain about one pound a year from an ideal weight in their mid-twenties. As you get older you require less food, because your metabolic rate – your body's ability to burn up fat for energy – slows down. Few people take account of this in their eating habits, however, so many 30–40 year olds can be as much as 15 pounds overweight. They no longer look so good and they see themselves as fat. Often, by the time they come to a Y class, they have tried every advertised diet going.

In general, the demands made on our eating habits by society are high. Sharing food or drink is a demonstration of friendship and our social lives centre round calorie intake – from cups of coffee to elaborate meals. In the street, in shops and on television, tempting taste sensations are always on display.

Barbara was 21 pounds overweight and most of that was around her hips and thighs. She had spent seven years trying a succession of crash diets: a grapefruit diet, high protein, low fat, calorie controlled, high carbohydrate. . . . Because she could never stick to them permanently, she always put the weight back on and eventually the struggle became too much. For Barbara, the Y was the last resort. She began a Y exercise programme and now she maintains her ideal weight.

One of the problems of dieting is that you do not lose fat

alone, you also lose water and lean body tissue, or muscle. This muscle you are losing is what enables you to look shapely and firm. Muscle is an active tissue and uses up energy, therefore the overall loss caused by dieting slows down your basic metabolic rate, the rate at which your body uses energy to maintain itself at rest. Therefore, when you reduce your calorie intake your body adapts to conserve energy and it functions on fewer calories. So if you diet and lose weight, then stop dieting and put the weight back on, it becomes twice as hard to lose it again because your body still only uses up a lower quantity of calories, leaving the surplus as fat for you to carry around. The bonus for Barbara is that in changing shape by exercise she now looks far better than when she lost weight by dieting and she has a good, well-proportioned body shape that is no longer bottom-heavy. Not everyone has a weight problem, however.

Peter joined the Y at 35, when he weighed exactly the same as he had in his early twenties. Because he had not been active since his school days, though, he had lost muscle and a much larger proportion of his body weight now consisted of fat. This meant that he had lost the body shape of his youth.

The big difference between a man in his twenties and a man in his forties is muscle. Most people, unless they do

something about it, lose about half their muscle mass between the ages of 18 and 65. This gradual atrophy is one of the most obvious signs of ageing and one which the Y Plan programme can help to slow down.

Following the Y Plan meant that Peter has not only maintained his constant weight but has also regained his muscular body shape. Remember, dieting alone does nothing for the muscles, which are what give you a good body shape. Exercise tones and firms muscles and helps to reduce fat, as many people like Barbara and Peter have been delighted to discover.

As teachers of exercise we have watched individual personal development with fascination. Time and again members of our exercise classes have achieved their individual goals, but more importantly their outlooks on life have changed. Like Barbara and Peter, they have gained some control over their lifestyles and the confidence to be, do and achieve what they want.

Not everybody, though, has a particular reason for wanting to exercise and it can be harder for such people to believe in and maintain the exercise habit. But a habit it must be – a habit so regular that to miss it feels strange, just like not brushing your teeth. When you don't brush your teeth, you feel bad and they deteriorate. When you don't exercise, you and your body are similarly affected.

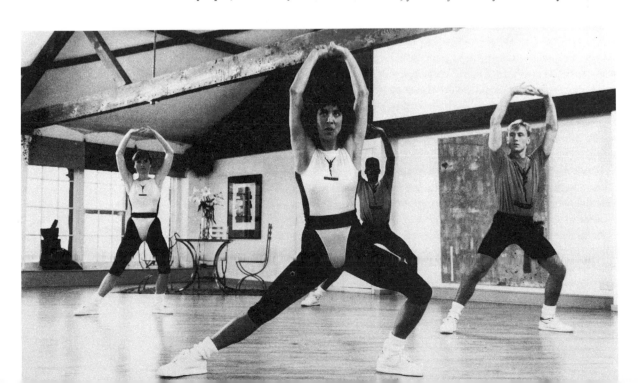

A physically fitter body will function much more efficiently for everything. Everyday tasks are easier to perform and mental agility is increased, but the benefits go deeper: *the likelihood of injury, illness and disease will decrease in a fit body, as do the effects of ageing.*

These long-term benefits are clearly just as significant as more obvious and visible effects like improving your body shape. But the mind and body adapt to and come to terms with inactivity with great ease and people don't always face up to the consequences of a sedentary lifestyle. They are reluctant to accept that a possible heart attack or immobility in a 70-year-old could well have been *prevented* by regular exercise. Another factor in the way we function and protect our body against physical and mental stress is a healthy diet. If we do not follow the essential ground rules of what, when and how much we eat, our bodies can suffer in much the same way as they do from lack of activity.

The Y Plan exercises are arranged on three levels – the second is a bit more demanding than the first, and so on. For those people who expect the Y Plan programme to keep them in shape, Levels 1–3 will achieve all that is necessary. Because most people will begin the Y Plan at Level 1, every exercise in that section is fully illustrated; in Levels 2 and 3 all new exercises are illustrated, but some of those which repeat an exercise learned earlier are referred back to the appropriate page for a photograph – though by that stage, you probably won't need one.

The exercises in Levels 1–3 consist of twelve-minute blocks centred on muscle-toning exercises (T) or aerobic exercises (A) – the idea is that the Y Plan alternates these in your exercise programme to ensure that your whole body is properly exercised. At the top of each page of exercises you will see the letter T or A within a circle, indicating which block you are in. (T and A appear together when you are doing exercises which relate to *both* blocks.)

Between each level there are transitional stages. These allow you gradually to progress to the next level. People generally find they are better at the muscle-toning exercises than the aerobic, or vice versa, at some stage, so transitional stages can combine exercises of either type from a higher level while you get used to the gradual increase in effort.

In many Y classes we exercise to music, choosing rhythms that are right for the pace of each exercise and that encourage people to get in the swing of things and keep moving. You can just as easily play your own choice of music or buy an inexpensive metronome from a music shop, and set the tempo to about 60 beats per minute (when each count will take 1 second). You can set it slightly faster or slower to suit you.

Each twelve-minute exercise block has a warm-up and a cool-down section. The warm-up is designed to loosen all the major joints of the body, to warm and stretch the muscles so that the body is prepared for the harder exercise session. The cool-down is designed to give the body time to recover from the workout. Its exercises are relaxed and slow and really stretch out all the muscles to minimise any after-effects of stiffness or muscle soreness.

As an integral part of the Y Plan, a number of fitness self-tests are included. The first one you must participate in comes after completing Level 1 for one week. Throughout this week, you will need to enter your performance record in the Y Plan diary (see p. 140), after your exercise sessions. (Instructions on how to enter your performance record are given in Chapter 3.) Then you repeat the fitness test after every six weeks of exercise. This will give you independent, accurate information as to how your body has adapted to muscle-toning, stretching and aerobic exercises, and will help you plan your progress towards a fitter, firmer, more shapely body. Throughout the book, stage by stage, we explain how you can get the best out of the Y Plan.

If up to now you've been wary about taking that first step to fitness, let the Y Plan guide you through fun, safe, progressive exercise programmes that set you realistic, tailor-made goals.

Y is for You.

Chapter One

THE Y PLAN AND FITNESS

The Y Plan is about fitness, *your* fitness. The first stage towards achieving fitness is to consider what we believe the term 'fitness' really means.

TOTAL FITNESS

In any one person this is a complex mixture of elements. It refers not only to your whole body, but includes every factor that affects healthy and enjoyable living. The state of a person's health has to be taken into account, as does their diet, or nutritional well-being. Related to these, and equally important, are emotional balance and social ease.

PHYSICAL FITNESS

Whatever the present states of your health and of your social and emotional life, these are related to your physical fitness, which is what the Y Plan is all about. Physical

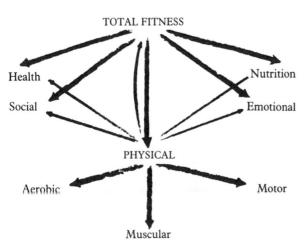

fitness includes the heart and lungs (aerobic fitness), strength and endurance of the muscles, flexibility of the joints and a reasonably low level of fat. Physical fitness relates to the ease with which you are able to carry out your daily activities and the amount of energy available to you. The fitter you are the more 'alive' you feel.

FEELING GOOD

The old maxim that a healthy body makes a healthy mind has been scientifically shown to contain a lot of truth. Regular exercise helps you in all sorts of ways to enjoy life more at every level.

Exercising may make you feel good at a psychological level because you've done something active or because you have achieved a goal or even because you've progressed further than before. It does get easier.

But exercise has a physiological effect on you too. The movement of exercise and its stimulation of the muscles cause showers of nerve impulses to stream into the brain, having an energising effect. You feel more animated and actually happier. Therapists are now using exercise as a treatment for depression and anxiety, and to promote emotional stability.

As well as pushing extra oxygen round the bloodstream, exercise stimulates the release of natural chemical substances in the body called endorphins, which also have the effect of making you feel good. Have you ever heard the term 'runner's high'? Well, endorphins and other chemicals are what cause this pleasurable feeling in athletes.

Don't worry! The Y Plan should become a habit but it won't become an addiction. It's just good to know that exercising sensibly not only improves your body, it really does make you feel better too.

BODY SHAPE

The Y Plan programme is to improve your body shape, to get you fit and help you feel happy with yourself.

In order to progress, you need to establish your own, realistic goals and not strive to achieve the impossible. The way to begin this is to look at what our individual bodies are capable of in terms of changing and improving.

Most of us have an idea of how we want to look, and for many of us our motives for starting out on the latest exercise or diet fad were to do with achieving that look and that shape. In reality, our own bodies determine our basic shape and structure and no workout or diet can change that. We can develop and improve, but none of us can turn into something we are not.

Before you start the Y Plan, then, it will help to know what body type you are, where you have excess fat and in what areas your muscles needs developing.

There are three basic categories of body type – Endomorphs, Mesomorphs and Ectomorphs. It is important to realise that not everyone fits perfectly into one of these categories but that we are likely to tend towards one of them, even though we may have some characteristics of the others.

ENDOMORPHS tend to be short, with wide hips and large proportions. They are usually rounded and covered by a layer of fairly evenly distributed body fat. They gain weight easily.

MESOMORPHS are broad-shouldered and narrow-waisted, with thick bones, and are generally athletic-looking.

ECTOMORPHS are long and lean, with narrow shoulders and hips. They have very little muscle bulk and are often thin, though they can become overweight.

Now we come to the difficult bit where you have to be really honest with yourself. Remove all your clothes and view your body in a full-length mirror. Try to determine your basic body type. Write down immediately all the characteristics you can identify that are part of your basic body structure. Come to terms with the difference between your actual and your desired body shape. Women normally store fat on thighs, buttocks, hips and bust. Other major fat stores can be the stomach and the back of the upper arm and shoulders. Men tend to store fat on their stomach and hips, but they too can store fat in the same places as women.

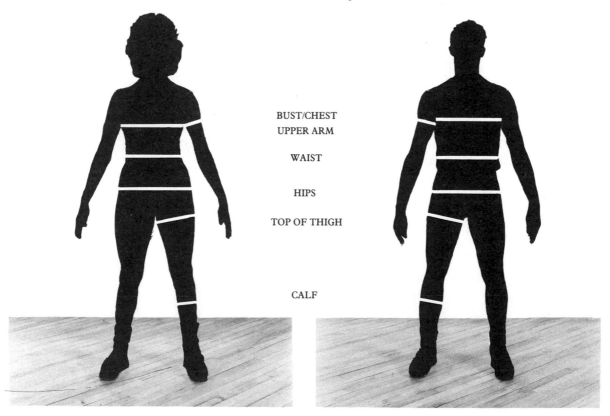

BUST/CHEST
UPPER ARM

WAIST

HIPS

TOP OF THIGH

CALF

The next stage is to view your body more closely. Where is your body fat? How is it affecting the shape of your body? What do you not like about yourself? What can you realistically do to change it? Make sure you view yourself critically from the front, the back and the sides, standing as you would normally do. Get into the habit of viewing your body regularly and you will be able to evaluate your changing shape by careful observation. It can also be useful to take measurements and then check changes in them. Take the largest measurement around the parts of the body shown opposite. If men measure more round the waist than round the hips, the risk of heart attack is doubled.

You can also weigh yourself after your first fitness test but don't weigh and measure yourself again until the next six-week fitness assessment. Weigh and measure a third time after the twelve-week test, and so on. It is important to understand, however, that you may not lose weight, because although you will be losing body fat it will be replaced by shapely muscle, which is heavier than body fat. One way to illustrate this is to realise that an ounce of butter will float on water but an ounce of steak will sink. Your measurement ratio, too, should change in relation to your fitness, so some measurements may increase rather than decrease, and this is perfectly acceptable.

As you look at your body shape regularly, you will also learn to evaluate your posture. Though you may not at first be aware of what is correct posture, as you do the exercises you will notice that your posture and body management improve and develop.

Never lose sight of your basic body type and its limitations. This will allow you to appreciate how you look and to value your own self-image.

Before taking part in a regular exercise programme, always be sure that you are in the right physical condition. To help you judge this, fill in the Y Plan questionnaire. If you are still in any doubt, consult your doctor.

Read the following questions carefully and answer as accurately as you can.

If you have answered 'Yes' to one or more questions, consult your doctor prior to starting a graduated exercise programme.

If you have answered 'No' to all questions, this is a reasonable assurance that it is safe for you to begin a graduated exercise programme.

	YES	NO
1 Has your doctor ever said you have heart disease, high blood pressure or any other cardiovascular problem?	....	....
2 Is there a history of heart disease in your family?	....	....
3 Do you ever have pains in your heart and chest, especially associated with minimal effort?	....	....
4 Do you often get headaches, feel faint or dizzy?	....	....
5 Do you suffer from either pain or limited movement in any joints which has been caused by exercise or might be aggravated with exercise?	....	....
6 Are you taking drugs/medication at the moment or recuperating from a recent illness or operation?	....	....
7 Are you pregnant?	....	....
8 Are you unaccustomed to exercise and aged over 50?	....	....
9 Do you have any other medical condition which you think may affect your ability to participate in exercise?	....	....

PLANNING AND PREPARATION

Here are some tips to help you get the best out of the Y Plan.

• Find a time in the day that becomes your exercise time – and stick with it.

• Make sure the time you choose doesn't compete with anyone else's needs.

• Make sure that family or flatmates know you are not available at your exercise time.

• Plan ahead. If an important engagement clashes with your exercise time, either find another time on that day for the Y Plan or choose another day but at your usual time. It is important to stick to your twelve minutes of exercise four times a week in order to build and maintain the exercise habit.

• Make room to do your exercise safely. Make sure there is no furniture to obstruct your movements.

• For floor exercises, make sure you have some kind of padded surface, such as a carpet, a towel or an exercise mat beneath you.

• Wear comfortable clothing, nothing tight or made of plastic materials and preferably something with a cotton base. For women, a good supporting bra is essential.

• Wear shoes with all-round support and sole cushioning or, if you prefer, at Levels 1 and 2, no shoes. Never exercise in socks. Good shoes are essential at Level 3.

• If you don't feel well, DO NOT EXERCISE. Pick it up another day. This applies even if you have a cold.

• The Y Plan should never be painful – if anything hurts, stop!

• Never hold your breath while exercising. A good general rule is to breathe out on the effort or as you go into a stretch. Breathing should otherwise be regular, relaxed and natural. There is no need to control it further.

• Don't exercise too soon after eating a heavy meal. This means wait about two hours before you begin your workout.

• Drink a little water while exercising if you need to.

• If you go away on holiday/business or get ill and do not do your Y Plan exercises for a week, drop back to your previous level for one week. If you miss two or three weeks of exercise, drop back to your previous level for two weeks.

• Try and do the Y Plan with a friend or partner.

• If an exercise doesn't feel comfortable, check the instructions again. Do it in a mirror or try to get someone else to watch and see if you are doing it correctly. If you still feel uncomfortable, try the alternative exercise where provided, or simply DON'T DO IT.

• Don't rush it. Be prepared to learn the exercises correctly.

• Note your progress on your performance record (see p. 140) so as to check that you are progressing as planned.

• Don't get disheartened if you don't go on improving as fast as you did at first. Don't worry. This is a quite normal reaction. Keep working and you will soon start improving again.

• Concentrate on *what* and *how* you are working, so that you exercise *effectively* and *safely*.

• Don't expect your first attempts at exercise to be effortless. If you feel that some of what you are doing is too hard, don't give up hope. Starting is the hardest part and you have already done that. Try to remember what you are doing for your body and why.

Chapter Two

HOW THE Y PLAN WORKS

The Y Plan is structured for you to work out four times each week, with one clear rest day each week when you don't exercise. As you get into the habit of this routine you will find yourself becoming fitter and more shapely, but if ever you find four sessions a week too much for you, remember that whatever exercise you can manage is better than none at all, and will help you to keep trim. If you cannot exercise four times a week, try to structure some definite frequency rather than fitting a session in only when you can find time. Fitness cannot be stored and without *regular* bouts of exercise, any gains the body makes are quickly lost.

A survey in *Physician and Sports Science Medicine* (July 1989) found that 50 per cent of people who took up some form of regular exercise had given it up within a year. But keeping a record of your own progress will help to motivate you in maintaining the exercise habit and seeing the regular improvements in your body shape and fitness that your records reveal will encourage you to keep going and even to aim for higher goals.

You will find, too, that the structure of the Y Plan – its simple but effective programme for moving up through the four levels and its carefully designed transitional stages – will act as a series of goals in itself. As you find yourself able to meet new challenges in the different levels, your commitment to your exercise habit will increase, as will your enjoyment also. With the Y Plan, working out is fun.

Every kind of exercise programme, no matter how simple, should incorporate a warm-up and a cool-down section for safety and effectiveness.

WARM-UP

The warm-up exercises protect the muscles, joints and heart from doing too much too soon and so prevent the risk of injury. These exercises have two elements (mobility/pulse-raising and stretching) which combine to ensure that you are physically and mentally prepared for your Y Plan workout at whatever level you have reached.

MOBILITY AND PULSE-RAISING   These exercises make up the first part of each warm-up section. Mobility exercises are designed to loosen up the joints used in the workout. The aim is to move each joint slowly and thoroughly throughout its full range. This stimulates more fluid in the joint and promotes easier movement and shock absorption. Pulse-raising exercises consist of large, rhythmic movements. Their scale and frequency put greater demands on the muscles, which therefore require more oxygen, and as the muscles (including the heart) work harder, heat is generated and released, literally warming up the body.

When performing mobility and pulse-raising exercises, check that you:

□ *Keep the correct posture described on pp. 134–5*

□ *Take the joint slowly through its full range of movement, keeping the movement smooth, and not jerky*

STRETCHING   The second sequence for the warm-up involves stretching and preparing all the major muscle groups to be used in the workout. Muscles are able to stretch and lengthen better after the warming process. Without it, not only will the results of the exercise be less effective but actual damage can occur. In the Y Plan warm-ups, you are given some different stretching exercises to perform before the muscle-toning exercises and the aerobic exercises.

As you progress in fitness through the Y Plan, you will find that the warm-up exercise sequences will become more rhythmic and continuous.

COOL-DOWN

These slow, relaxed exercises allow the body time to recover from its workout. When the muscles have worked

WARM-UP

MOBILITY AND

PULSE RAISING

*for muscle toning
and aerobics*

WARM-UP

STRETCHING

for muscle toning

WARM-UP

STRETCHING

for aerobics

TONING

EXERCISES

COOL-DOWN

*for muscle toning
and aerobics*

AEROBIC

EXERCISES

hard they are shortened and tight, and stretching them out in the cool-down returns them to their original length and reduces their tension, easing subsequent stiffness or soreness.

After the workout, too, the muscles are at their warmest so it is an ideal time to improve your flexibility by holding and developing the stretch positions for longer. You can increase the length of the cool-down exercises according to your own comfort and the time you have available.

To help loosen up the body and get the circulation going again after prolonged stretches it is also a good idea, if you have time, to do some more mobility and pulse-raising exercises, but always keeping them slow and controlled for the cool-down.

To stretch muscles safely, both in the warm-up and the cool-down, always remember:

> □ *Never stretch a cold muscle*
>
> □ *Take time to find a comfortable position and gently ease into it and out of it at the end*
>
> □ *Once you feel the stretch on the muscle, stop and hold the position quite still. If it feels uncomfortable, change positions*
>
> □ *Never bounce or push in stretching exercises*
>
> □ *The pulling sensation should be felt in the bulky part of the muscle. If the muscle shakes, you have gone too far*
>
> □ *Don't force your knees backwards in any leg-muscle stretch or lock your elbows in shoulder stretches*

YOUR PERSONAL Y PLAN – WHAT'S IN IT

Apart from warm-up and cool-down, here is a guide to what you can expect to find generally within each level and block of the Y Plan.

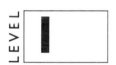

BLOCK T – (MUSCLE TONING)
6 minutes

These exercises improve muscle strength, endurance and shape.

The following parts of the body are worked: front and back of legs, buttocks, stomach, chest, upper arms.

The slow speed of the exercises allows you time to gain the correct exercise technique, vital for Level 1. Your muscles will not gain full benefit if these exercises are not performed correctly, and there is also the possibility of muscle or joint injury.

BLOCK A – (AEROBIC)
6 minutes

These exercises make up a sequence that is rhythmic and flowing, making the lungs and circulatory system work harder in order to deliver oxygen to enable the muscles to cope with sustained activity.

BLOCK T – (MUSCLE TONING)
6 minutes

The same parts of the body are worked as in Level 1/Block T, with additional exercise for the inside and outside of the thighs. The number of times the exercises are performed has been increased. The speed of some exercises is also slightly quicker.

BLOCK A – (AEROBIC)
6 minutes

Some exercises from Level 1/Block A are repeated and new ones are added. They are performed with increased intensity and the size of the movements is also enlarged. The combination of exercise is more demanding, and more taxing of motor fitness (co-ordination).

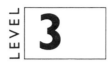

BLOCK T – (MUSCLE TONING)
7½ minutes

The same parts of the body are worked, but using new and varied exercises. The number of exercise repetitions has been increased and the sequence of exercises is continuous. Because the exercises have become more difficult, continue to review and check your exercise technique.

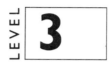

BLOCK A – (AEROBIC)
7½ minutes

Exercises have become increasingly demanding in intensity and duration, and in their complexity.

All the aerobic exercises have their own techniques and will not be effective if performed incorrectly (quite apart from the problems of injury). If you think the programme appears too easy, double-check how you are performing the exercises. We have found that even highly fit exercisers can become breathless from Level 1/Block A.

Now you know the basics of what is in the Y Plan programme. Because it's better to understand as much as possible about fitness, we have included more detailed information about muscle groups and posture and how exercise affects them at the back of the book (see p. 133).

Chapter Three

BEGINNING
THE Y PLAN

ASSESSMENT

In order to determine the level at which you start the Y Plan we recommend strongly that you follow the Y Plan assessment. Everyone should complete Level 1 for one week (as below):

MONDAY	T BLOCK	X
TUESDAY		
WEDNESDAY	BLOCK A	O
THURSDAY		
FRIDAY	T BLOCK	X
SATURDAY		
SUNDAY	BLOCK A	O

After you have exercised each day you should enter your performance record in your Y Plan diary, on page 140, referring to the information on this page and the next for guidance. Your completed diary at the end of the week should look something like the example above.

MUSCLE TONING BLOCKS

FILL IN '0' IF YOU WERE STRUGGLING, UNCOMFORTABLE, HARD WORKED

- Unable to do the exercises properly
- Working muscles have a burning sensation
- Working muscles feel like jelly
- Need to stop, cannot complete the routine
- 24–48 hours later muscles and joints ache

or

FILL IN 'X' IF YOU WERE CHALLENGED BUT COULD COPE

- Able to perform the exercises but with a lot of effort
- Muscles get warm and tired
- Just able to finish the routine
- 24–48 hours later muscles feel a little sore

or

FILL IN '√' IF YOU MANAGED EASILY

- Able to perform the exercises with ease and without concentration
- Muscles do not feel that they are having to work against any resistance
- At the end of the routine you are ready for more exercise
- 24–48 hours later no sign of muscles having been worked at all

CHOOSING YOUR Y PLAN LEVEL

You now have to interpret the result that you recorded in your diary in order to determine your starting level on the Y Plan.

If most or all of your scores were '0' or 'X' rated start carefully at Level 1.

AEROBIC BLOCKS

FILL IN '0' IF YOU WERE STRUGGLING, UNCOMFORTABLE, HARD WORKED

- Have difficulty breathing
- Feel very hot
- Unable to do the exercises properly
- Feel dizzy
- Legs feel like jelly
- Need to stop
- 24–48 hours later you still feel fatigued

or

FILL IN 'X' IF YOU WERE CHALLENGED BUT COULD COPE

- Breathing heavily
- Feel very warm
- Able to do the exercises but have to concentrate
- Legs work hard to keep going
- Ready to stop by the end of the routine
- Soon recover immediately after exercise

or

FILL IN '√' IF YOU MANAGED EASILY

- Little or no increase in breathing rate
- Don't feel much warmer
- Exercises performed with little thought
- No real effort required by legs
- Need to work for longer

If most of your scores were '√' rated, then start at transition Level 1/2.

If all of your scores were '√' rated, then start at Level 2 for one week. If your scores show a majority of '√'s and you are coping easily with all the exercises, go on to transitional Level 2/3.

You now know at which level to start the Y Plan. In addition you have learnt to perform the exercises correctly and safely in order to minimise the possibility of strain or injury – and there are variations of these exercises at all levels.

Your next step is to take the Y Plan fitness test (see page 20).

THE Y PLAN FITNESS TEST

This test (on p. 20) enables you to determine your present level of fitness. The same test is used as a regular check every six weeks so that you can evaluate your progress. Comparison of results from subsequent fitness tests will only be significant if you ensure that you always do the exercises in exactly the same way.

The fitness test is made up of muscle fitness exercises and aerobic exercises, both of which test your motor fitness (co-ordination) too.

All of us, at some time or another, have been curious to find out just how fit we really are. Remember, though, to beware of the term 'normal' in terms of fitness tests. It is usually a mistake to compare yourself to so-called 'average' or 'normal' levels of fitness, and even more of a mistake to compare yourself with athletes or sports stars. Improvements should be measured in terms of your own 'norms', which the Y Plan fitness test will demonstrate for you.

It is very hard to standardise results within these tests, so comparing your results with other people's is not going to be of much use to you. Even so, we have incorporated tables of 'norms' devised from thousands of test results, so that you can get some idea of how your performance rates compared to that of the general population. Just remember that improvement within your own scores is by far the most important thing to watch for.

To get the most accurate results from your Y Plan fitness test, you must try to do the tests in exactly the same way each time, after one week, six weeks, twelve weeks and so on, and record your results in the table on p. 139. Remember, you must answer the Y Plan questionnaire about your general state of health before beginning any exercise programme.

FITNESS TEST

Timed Press-Ups

PURPOSE: TO TEST MUSCLE STRENGTH AND ENDURANCE   **1** *minute*

• Take up whichever of the three illustrated press-up positions is more suitable for you. Men are expected to choose from only the last two

• Ensure that your hands are just wider than shoulder-width apart and immediately beneath your shoulders. Remember this position in order to repeat it as exactly as possible the next time you do the fitness test

• Hold your stomach in tightly and tilt your pelvis correctly so as not to allow your back to hollow

• Set your alarm or timer for one minute and begin, counting each full repetition

• With each press-up your forehead should touch the floor and your arms should be fully extended. With the intermediate and full press-ups, your thighs, stomach and chest must also touch the floor

• Breathe steadily – choose a pattern that fits with every press-up and is comfortable for you

Record the maximum number of press-ups you can perform correctly in one minute. You must not count any press-ups that do not go all the way down or all the way up. Check your score against the following 'norms' and record it on p. 139.

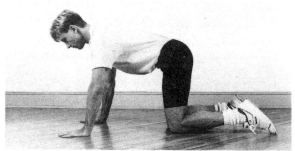

Box Press-Up Level 1

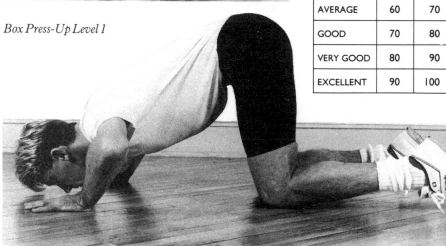

PRESS-UPS/WOMEN BEGINNER						
	21	21–30	31–40	41–50	51–60	61–70
VERY POOR	30	40	30	20	10	5
POOR	40	50	40	30	20	10
FAIR	50	60	50	40	30	20
AVERAGE	60	70	60	50	40	30
GOOD	70	80	70	60	50	40
VERY GOOD	80	90	80	70	60	50
EXCELLENT	90	100	90	80	70	60

PRESS-UPS/WOMEN INTERMEDIATE					
	21	21–30	31–40	41–50	51–60	61–70
VERY POOR	15	20	15	10	7	4
POOR	20	25	20	15	10	7
FAIR	25	30	25	18	13	10
AVERAGE	30	35	30	22	17	12
GOOD	35	40	35	25	20	15
VERY GOOD	40	45	40	30	25	20
EXCELLENT	45	50	45	35	30	25

PRESS-UPS/MEN INTERMEDIATE					
	21	21–30	31–40	41–50	51–60	61–70
VERY POOR	15	25	20	15	12	9
POOR	20	30	25	20	15	12
FAIR	25	35	30	23	18	15
AVERAGE	30	40	35	27	22	17
GOOD	35	47	42	32	27	22
VERY GOOD	40	55	50	40	35	30
EXCELLENT	45	65	60	50	45	40

Intermediate Press-Up

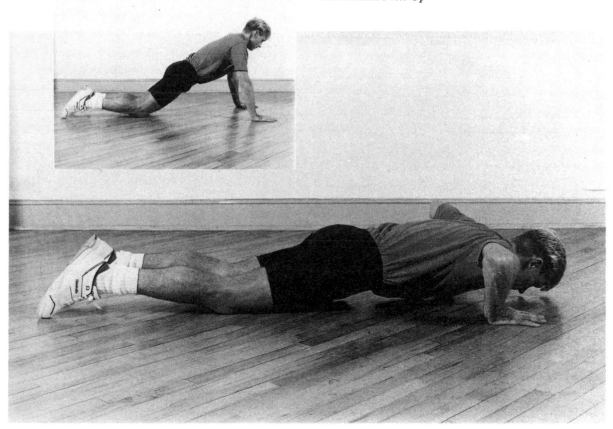

PRESS - UPS / WOMEN FULL						
	21	21–30	31–40	41–50	51–60	61–70
VERY POOR	10	12	10	7	5	3
POOR	13	15	13	10	7	5
FAIR	15	19	15	13	10	7
AVERAGE	20	23	20	15	13	10
GOOD	24	27	24	20	15	13
VERY GOOD	27	30	27	23	20	17
EXCELLENT	30	35	30	26	23	20

PRESS - UPS / MEN FULL						
	21	21–30	31–40	41–50	51–60	61–70
VERY POOR	10	15	10	7	5	3
POOR	13	20	13	10	7	5
FAIR	15	25	15	13	10	7
AVERAGE	20	30	20	15	13	10
GOOD	24	37	24	20	15	13
VERY GOOD	27	45	27	23	20	17
EXCELLENT	30	55	30	26	23	20

Full Press-Up

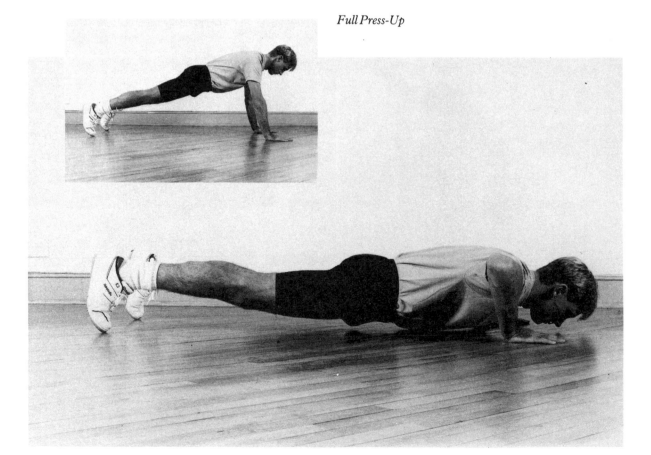

FITNESS TEST

Sit and Reach

PURPOSE: TO TEST FOR
SUPPLENESS

This should be performed when your body is warm.

● Lay out a tape measure as shown, and secure it at the 15 inch mark with a piece of sticky tape

● Sit, as in the photograph, placing your heels on the sticky tape about 10 inches apart with your toes pointing up to the ceiling

● Curl your trunk forwards and reach your hands as far towards (or beyond) your heels as possible. Don't bounce or jerk as this can cause damage to muscles or the lower back and does not measure genuine suppleness

● At the furthest point you can reach, hold still for a count of three. Where your finger reaches on the tape at the end of this count is your score

Record your best three attempts, check them against these 'norms' and complete your fitness test record on p. 139.

	UNDER 35	36–45	46+
	WOMEN		
EXCELLENT	23″	23″	22″
GOOD	21″	21″	19″
AVERAGE	18″	17″	15″
FAIR	14″	12″	11″
POOR	11″	10″	9″
	MEN		
EXCELLENT	21″	22″	20″
GOOD	19″	19″	17″
AVERAGE	15″	14″	13″
FAIR	10″	11″	9″
POOR	7″	5″	5″

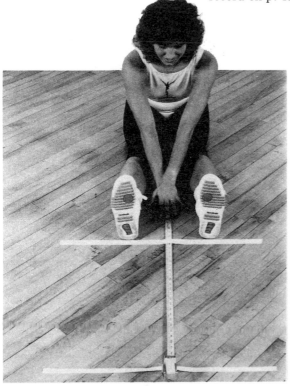

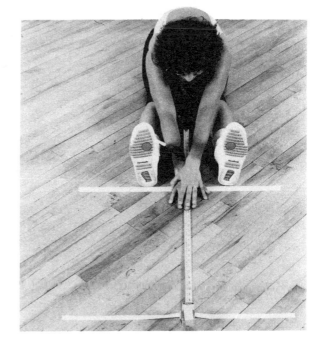

FITNESS TEST

Either

Timed Curl-Ups (Moderate)

PURPOSE: TO TEST
MUSCLE STRENGTH AND
ENDURANCE   1 minute
....

- Lie on your back with both knees bent so that your feet are 1–2 feet away from your buttocks

- Place one hand behind your head to support it and prevent neck ache. Reach the other hand down to rest on your thigh

- Curl your head and shoulders off the floor so that the hand on your leg slides up until your middle finger reaches the centre of the knee cap

- Return to lying down with your hand back on your thigh. Your shoulders must touch the floor fully but the head does not need to

Or

Timed Curl-Ups (Hard)

PURPOSE: TO TEST
MUSCLE STRENGTH AND
ENDURANCE   1 minute
....

- Lie on your back with both knees bent, so that your feet are 1–2 feet away from your buttocks, with your head slightly off the floor

- Place both hands with fingertips behind the ears for support

- Curl head and shoulders off the floor until your elbows touch your mid-thighs

- Return to start with your shoulder blades fully on the floor

- If you find you are top-heavy and your feet always come off the floor, get someone to hold behind your heels so you can pull in against this as you sit up. Securing the feet any other way changes the exercise too much

> □ *Tilt your pelvis to keep your lower back pushed into the floor*
>
> □ *Keep your stomach flat throughout the movement*
>
> □ *Be sure not to jerk up or pull on your head as this could damage your neck*
>
> □ *Breathe regularly: out as you go up, in as you go down. Do not hold your breath.*

CURL-UPS / WOMEN
MODERATE

	21	21–30	31–40	41–50	51–60	61–70
VERY POOR	35	40	35	30	25	20
POOR	40	45	40	35	30	25
FAIR	45	50	45	40	35	30
AVERAGE	50	55	50	45	40	35
GOOD	55	60	55	50	45	40
VERY GOOD	60	65	60	55	50	45
EXCELLENT	65	70	65	60	55	50

CURL-UPS / MEN
MODERATE

	21	21–30	31–40	41–50	51–60	61–70
VERY POOR	35	45	40	35	28	23
POOR	40	50	45	40	38	33
FAIR	45	55	50	45	38	33
AVERAGE	50	60	55	50	43	38
GOOD	55	67	62	57	50	45
VERY GOOD	60	75	70	65	58	53
EXCELLENT	65	80	75	70	63	58

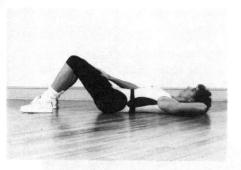

When you have practised once or twice to get the exercise right, set your alarm/cooking timer for one minute and do the exercise as many times as you can in a controlled manner, counting the times and remembering to ensure that your free hand reaches the top of your knee or your elbows reach mid-thighs every time. Record your score on p. 139 and check it against the appropriate 'norm' chart shown here.

Moderate Curl-Up

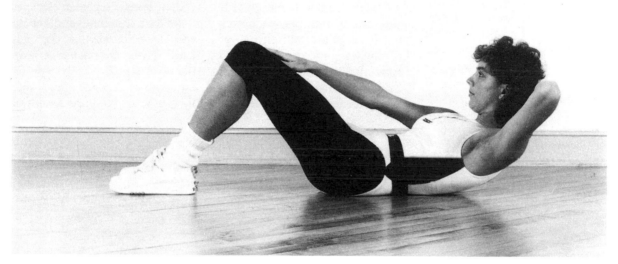

CURL-UPS/WOMEN HARD						
	21	21–30	31–40	41–50	51–60	61–70
VERY POOR	15	20	15	13	8	3
POOR	20	25	20	15	10	5
FAIR	25	30	25	20	15	10
AVERAGE	30	35	30	25	20	15
GOOD	35	40	35	30	25	20
VERY GOOD	40	45	40	35	30	25
EXCELLENT	45	50	45	40	35	30

CURL-UPS/MEN HARD						
	21	21–30	31–40	41–50	51–60	61–70
VERY POOR	15	25	20	18	13	8
POOR	20	30	25	20	15	10
FAIR	25	35	30	25	20	15
AVERAGE	30	40	35	30	25	20
GOOD	35	47	42	37	32	27
VERY GOOD	40	55	50	45	40	35
EXCELLENT	45	65	60	55	50	45

FITNESS TEST

Timed Step-Ups

PURPOSE: TO TEST
AEROBIC FITNESS

For this you need to measure your pulse after exercise. To do this correctly, find the pulse on the thumb side of the wrist with the fingers (not the thumb) of the other hand. You will find it increasingly easier with experi-ence, so practise before you begin the fitness test and record how many beats there are in 30 seconds. Then:

● Make yourself a step wide enough for both feet that is strong and stable and between 16 inches and 20 inches high. A chair or a stool will do

● Using a metronome (which you can buy quite cheaply from a music shop) set yourself one of the following speeds: 60 beats, 80 beats, 100 beats, 120 beats. The higher the setting, the harder the test. Remember, even if you think you're fit, it's better to begin gently

● Practise stepping up and down in time to the beat – right foot up then left foot up, left foot down then right foot down. Straighten both legs at the top before step-ping down

● Start the metronome at your chosen speed, set your clock or timer for five minutes and step up and down in rhythm for that long. If you are unable to keep the rhythm going, keep stepping for about 15 seconds after losing it, then stop. Note the length of

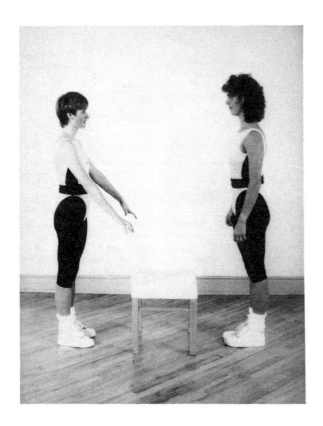

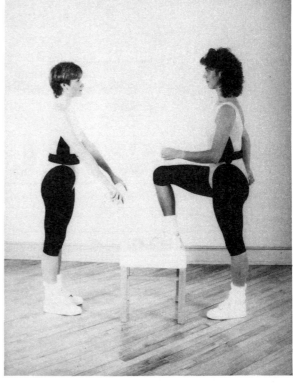

time you exercised, in seconds

• Sit down and begin to find your pulse. Wait one minute after stopping exercise, then count your pulse for the next 30 seconds, recording the number of beats on p. 139

• Calculate your aerobic fitness index. A bit of maths is required here. First, multiply the time *in seconds* that you stepped for by 100; this is to make the result into a reasonable whole number. Now multiply your pulse count by 5½. Lastly, divide the second figure into the first. The result is your

current fitness index score

The multiples are based on ratios established by scientific tests. Craig Sharp has used this method of aerobic fitness testing for over 20 years on people ranging from world champions to invalids. For example:

If you stepped for 5 minutes (300 seconds) $\times$ 100 = 30,000
If your pulse was 50 $\times$ 5½ = 275
Divide 30,000 by 275 = 108

This is your correct aerobic score and you are in the Very Good category.

Now compare your actual score with the following:

ATHLETES	140+
EXCELLENT	120–139
VERY GOOD	100–119
GOOD	80–99
FAIR	50–79
POOR	49 and lower

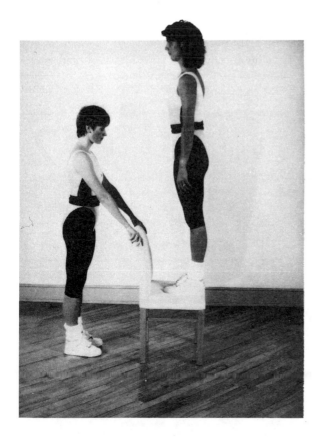

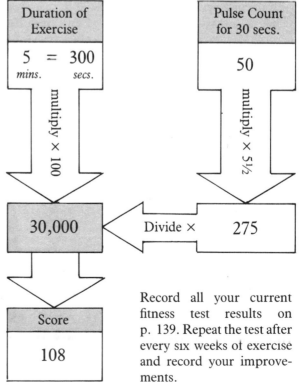

Duration of Exercise	Pulse Count for 30 secs.
5 = 300 *mins. secs.*	50
multiply $\times$ 100	multiply $\times$ 5½
30,000	Divide $\times$ 275
Score	
108	

Record all your current fitness test results on p. 139. Repeat the test after every six weeks of exercise and record your improvements.

THE Y PLAN DIARY

(See blank diary for you to complete on page 140)

You have now completed the Y Plan assessment and know at what level to begin. You have also completed the fitness test which is for comparative purposes only. You are now ready to find out about your Y Plan diary.

The example of the diary below illustrates how a level is followed for four weeks by alternating the toning and aerobic blocks throughout the week. Of course you could vary your exercise days from those shown, providing you still exercise on alternate days.

To assist your progress to a higher level, there are two transitional weeks between each level and the next. Each transitional week combines exercise blocks from both levels.

By filling in your Y Plan diary after every exercise session, in the same way that you recorded your assessment week, you will see, when you have a majority of ticks, that you are ready to move to a higher level.

In the first week of each level, most of the exercises should be a struggle. By Week Four of each level, the majority of the exercises should be much easier, indicating that you are ready to move on, and the transition stages should be little more of a challenge. In any progressive programme there will be times when you seem to stop improving. Don't worry if this happens. It is just a phase and you will soon continue to improve again.

The Y Plan can be flexible and it is designed to meet your needs. It may be that four weeks on one level is too long or even not long enough. As you can see in Jane's diary, she has not recorded a majority of ticks in Week Four. Consequently she should complete a further week or more at Level 1 until she does record a majority of ticks. Jane should now proceed to the transitional two weeks before progressing further to Level 2.

Once you have performed at Level 3 and the scores you have recorded in your diary indicate that the blocks have become easy (i.e. you have recorded a majority of '√'s), you can progress further by:

a. Alternating the muscle-toning and aerobic blocks for six days each week, allowing one day free from exercise.

or

b. Performing both blocks (24 minutes) of exercises for four days a week on alternate days.

L E V E L 1

Week / Date	BLOCK	ASSESS	1	2	3	4
MON	T		●	●	●	●
TUES						
WED	A		●	●	●	●
THURS						
FRI	T		●	●	●	●
SAT						
SUN	A		●	●	●	●

L E V E L 2

Week / Date	BLOCK	TRANSITION	1	2	3	4
MON	T	● ●	●	●	●	●
TUES						
WED	A	● ●	●	●	●	●
THURS						
FRI	T	● ●	●	●	●	●
SAT						
SUN	A	● ●	●	●	●	●

Remember even at this stage to continue completing your performance record and your fitness test every six weeks. (See appendix, pages 139–41.)

The results in your diary are only significant if you know exactly how to do the exercises and if you put all your effort into performing them.

When we described the broad content of each exercise block we stressed that unless you are doing the exercises correctly and with effort, they may seem too easy. It is also significant that some of you starting out on the Y Plan find Level 1 exercises easy for Week One, but having repeated them for a further week, you become familiar with the exercises and can put in more effort, and your body finds them more challenging.

As you progress through the levels you may be better at toning exercise than at aerobic exercise, or vice versa. Therefore it may be more appropriate to perform two different levels during the same week, as you would during a transitional stage. For example, if you have completed Level 2 but find the Level 3 aerobics block too difficult, you can move up to Level 3 toning but remain on Level 2 aerobics.

So don't always be in a hurry to move on to a higher level before you have given your body a chance to adapt to these new exercises. When you do move up, persevere as you did at the beginning: there will be some new difficulties but you progressed through the earlier exercises and you can do the same thing again.

Record your performance for every level because it will help you determine whether or not you are working on the right level. Remember that if you miss out on exercise due to illness, holiday, a business trip or whatever, your performance record will tell you whether or not you need to drop a level for a while to regain your previous fitness.

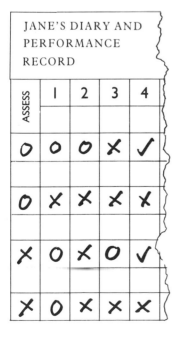

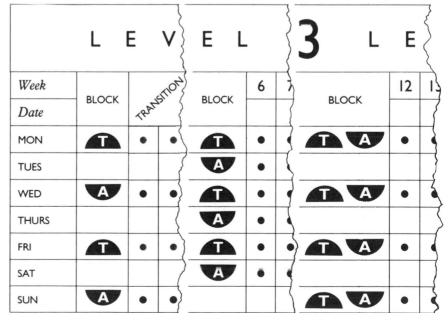

Chapter Four

THE Y PLAN EXERCISES

When you read through the exercises for all blocks you will see that the first line of each gives its name followed by the number of times you need to perform it, using right or left and moving forwards or backwards, and then we give the number of 'counts' each exercise will take to complete (indicated next to the metronome symbol).

At all levels you count 'one and', 'two and', 'three and' and so on and each such count takes about one second.

Some exercises may only take one 'count' to complete, others may take longer, using two, four, six, eight or more counts.

You can adjust the intensity of an exercise (making it easier or harder) by changing its tempo. You can make an exercise harder by speeding it up, but it can be more dangerous to exercise quickly as your control over your movements may be lost: sometimes, with speed, momentum takes over and the exercise becomes ineffective. Slowing an exercise down considerably can also make it more demanding and this can be a preferable way to increase your exertion as it ensures good control throughout the full range of movement.

When you feel confident that you can complete an exercise properly, you may feel you want to experiment by varying the speed slightly in order to feel the different demands made on you.

Once you have become familiar with the exercises, each block should not take longer than twelve minutes in total: the warm-up should last for three minutes, the muscular toning/aerobic exercises should take between six and seven-and-a-half minutes, and the cool-down should last from one-and-a-half to three minutes.

Either

EXERCISE   5A

Box Press-Ups
8

PURPOSE: TO STRENGTHEN THE MUSCLES IN THE BACK OF THE UPPER ARMS (TRICEPS) AND CHEST (PECTORALS)

16

- Come up on to all fours and place your hands with fingers

ing the elbows, don't snap them! (1 count)

- Do this 8 times

□ *Feel the arms working*

□ *Constantly check your position*

□ *Don't round the shoulders*

□ *Breathe regularly*

The second line of the exercise description in the warm-ups, cool-downs and toning exercises tells you its purpose and which muscles are being used to do what. (A detailed explanation with diagrams of the major muscle groups is given on p. 32.) All exercises in the aerobic blocks work the heart, lungs and circulatory system, and operate as a flowing sequence of exercises.

Throughout the blocks, some variations on basic

exercises are given, so if a particular position does not suit you, try an alternative which has the same purpose. The need to do this may not have anything to do with your level of fitness; it may be to do with individual body shape and personal preference – some exercise positions suit some people better than others.

Once you understand each block of exercises and how to do them, it may help you to use cue cards (see p. 142) to remember the routines.

The quality of the movements that make up the exercises is vital for achieving the results you want them to have. Always remember to:

□ *Isolate all your movements (that is, keep the rest of the body still and under control)*

□ *Think tall but relax your shoulders and keep your neck long*

□ *Be spatially aware – fully extend on every movement around the body, with control*

□ *Be aware of weight transference and balance*

□ *Take your weight through the whole foot when walking, marching or jogging. Move toe to heel when you are on the spot, making sure the heel is in contact with the floor. Move heel through to toe when you are moving along*

□ *Bend your knees and push your heels down on landing when performing high-impact (jumping or skipping) exercises*

□ *Breathe out on the effort*

EXPLAINING PELVIC TILT

Especially important for correct posture during exercise is the pelvic tilt.

● Place your hands on your hips with the thumbs pointing forwards and the fingers pointing back

● Stand with your feet shoulder-width apart and knees slightly bent

● Pull in your stomach muscles and tuck your buttocks under. Push down with your fingers and up with your thumbs as if you are tipping a basin towards you. This tilts the pelvis correctly and you will notice that the hollow curve in your lower back is reduced

● Now extend your legs, trying to maintain correct pelvic tilt. Your stomach should be flatter and your bottom tucked further under

Try the pelvic tilt side-on in front of a mirror to check that you are doing it correctly. It may take a little practice to master it.

There is reference to the pelvic tilt in many Y Plan exercise blocks so once you have mastered it standing, try it in other positions – box position (on all fours) or lying on your back.

EXPLAINING PELVIC FLOOR EXERCISE

The pelvic floor muscles are the muscle and tissue that form the base, or floor, of the pelvis. It is vital that these muscles maintain their tone to prevent the problem of stress incontinence.

The following exercise will work the pelvic floor and can be done at any time of the day. It should be done as frequently as possible and is important for men as well as women.

● Sit upright in a chair

● Slowly tighten and pull up the back and front passages (imagine you are drawing these muscles up inside to control the bladder and bowel)

● Hold for 3–5 counts

● Gradually release first the front then the back

● Don't hold your breath

Women should note that these muscles are particularly vulnerable during pregnancy because they support the weight of the baby and will naturally lose much of their tone. Therefore pelvic floor exercise *must* be performed frequently throughout pregnancy and with vigour immediately after childbirth.

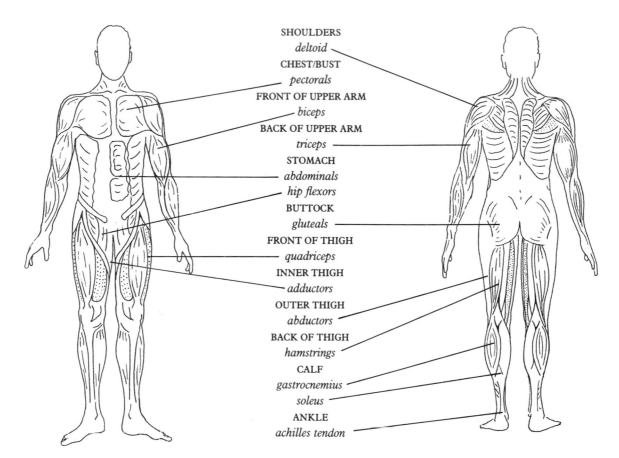

SHOULDERS
deltoid
CHEST/BUST
pectorals
FRONT OF UPPER ARM
biceps
BACK OF UPPER ARM
triceps
STOMACH
abdominals
hip flexors
BUTTOCK
gluteals
FRONT OF THIGH
quadriceps
INNER THIGH
adductors
OUTER THIGH
abductors
BACK OF THIGH
hamstrings
CALF
gastrocnemius
soleus
ANKLE
achilles tendon

EXPLAINING THE BODY'S MUSCLES

As you become familiar with the exercises you will recognise which muscles you are using. The illustration above shows you exactly where you have what; the muscle groups are the same for men and women.

POSITIVE OVERLOAD

When your physical activity becomes greater than your body can cope with in complete comfort – for instance, running some distance or climbing stairs fast – you will become a bit breathless and your muscles will begin to ache. This is because the body's systems are having to work harder than usual; the breathlessness and the aches signal that your body is trying to extend its capacity to cope with extra demands.

It is important not to get carried away with enthusiasm as you begin the Y Plan exercises and to think that the harder and faster you go the more good you will do. But

you do need to be aware of reaching the point where you no longer cope with ease during an exercise – a necessary aspect of effective exercise – and reaching that point of positive overload will help you through the levels of exercise. It is important not to push too far too soon, however, as this could result in you feeling tired, stiff or sore next day, and you might also feel deterred from carrying on!

As you graduate through the workouts you will realise that bit by bit it takes longer for you to tire or to become breathless. This means you are getting fitter.

EXERCISE ABBREVIATIONS			
R	= right	Fwds	= forwards
L	= left	S	= slowly
Bwds	= backwards	F	= fast

WARM - UP

The warm-up section is divided into two parts.

The first two-minutes are always done regardless of whether your main exercise block on a given day is for toning or aerobics.

You then follow this with one minute of stretching for either the toning warm-up or the aerobic warm-up. After completing the appropriate warm-up, you go on to six minutes of toning or aerobic exercise, followed by the three-minute cool-down.

Mobility and pulse-raising (for muscle toning and aerobics)

These exercises are to loosen the joints, to generate heat and warm the muscles. Remember always to check your posture and compare it with the photographs as you perform. Remember to count 'one and' as one second throughout Level 1.

2
minutes

EXERCISE   1

Shoulder Circles

2 Fwds + 2 Bwds

PURPOSE: TO MOBILISE
THE SHOULDERS

16

• Stand with feet shoulder-width apart and check your posture

• Circle both shoulders by rounding them forward, lifting them up, pulling them back to open the chest, then relaxing them down (4 counts)

• Do this twice forwards and twice backwards

□ *Make the movement as large as possible*

□ *Move smoothly*

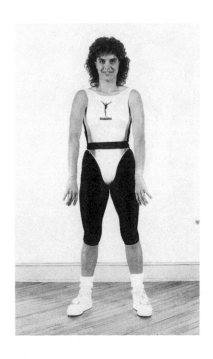
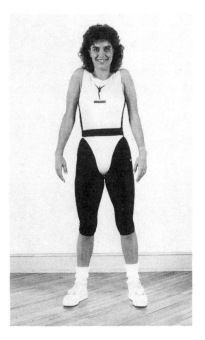
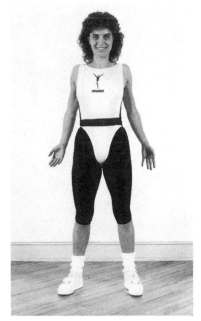

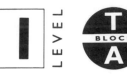

EXERCISE 2

Ankle Circles

4R + 4L

PURPOSE: TO MOBILISE
THE ANKLES

8

- Stand on the left leg, place the right toes on the floor near the left foot

- Circle the right ankle 4 times, taking it forwards then out, back and round (4 counts)

- Repeat this 4 times with the left ankle (4 counts)

☐ *Keep the hips still*

☐ *Feel the movement in the ankles*

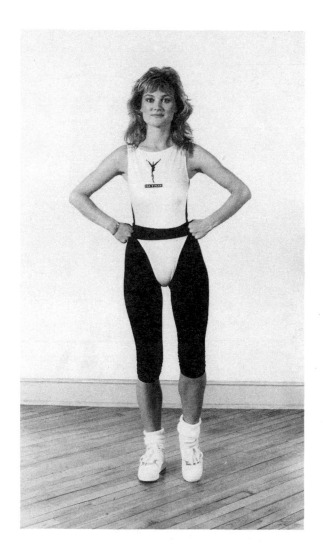

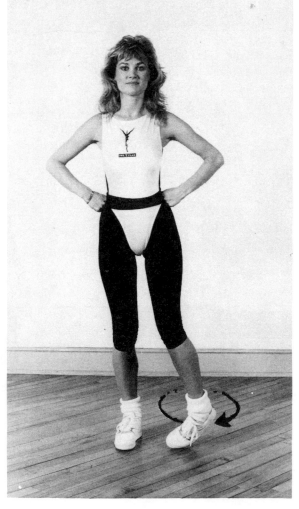

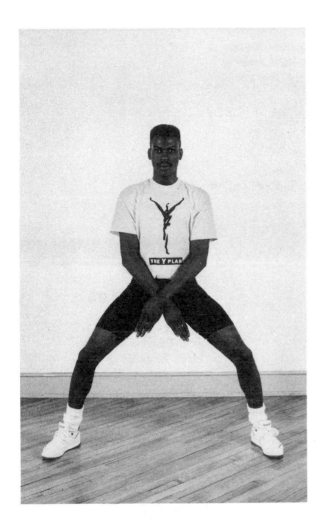

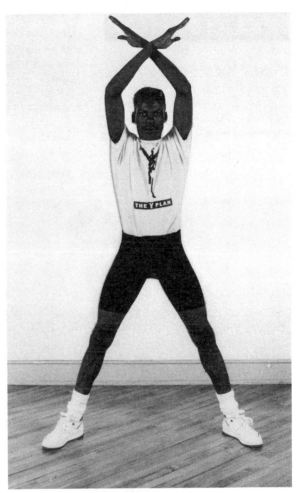

EXERCISE 3

Knee Bends and Arm Circles

8

PURPOSE: TO GENERATE
HEAT AND WARM THE
MUSCLES

16

● Stand with feet just over shoulder-width apart and toes pointing slightly out, with arms out sideways at shoulder-height

● Slowly bend the knees, swinging the arms down across in front of the body then up and out above the head as you straighten your legs (2 counts)

● Do this 8 times

☐ *Keep the back straight and the pelvis tucked under*

☐ *Push the knees out over the toes*

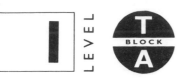

I LEVEL
T BLOCK
A

EXERCISE 4

Marches

16

PURPOSE: TO GENERATE
HEAT AND WARM THE
MUSCLES

16

- March on the spot, gradually lifting the knees a little higher and swinging your bent arms a little more vigorously (R + L = 1 count)

- Do this 16 times

☐ *Use a toe/heel action as your foot returns to the floor*

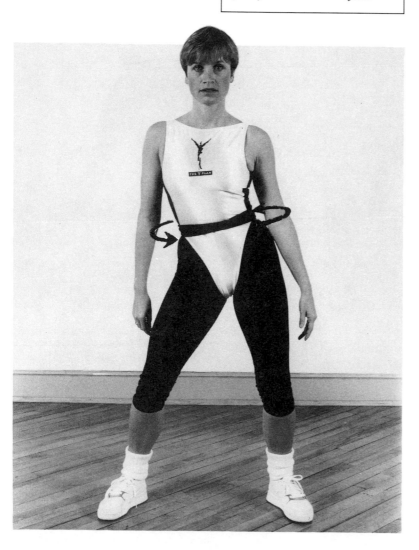

EXERCISE 5

Hip Circles

4R + 4L

PURPOSE: TO MOBILISE
THE LOWER BACK

16

- Stand with feet shoulder-width apart and knees slightly bent

- Circle the hips by taking them to the right, backwards, to the left, then forwards, using the stomach muscles (2 counts)

- Do this 4 times to the right and 4 to the left

☐ *Feel your stomach muscles assisting the movement*

☐ *Keep the knees slightly flexed and over your feet*

☐ *Keep the shoulders still*

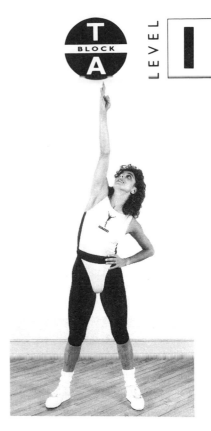

LEVEL **1**

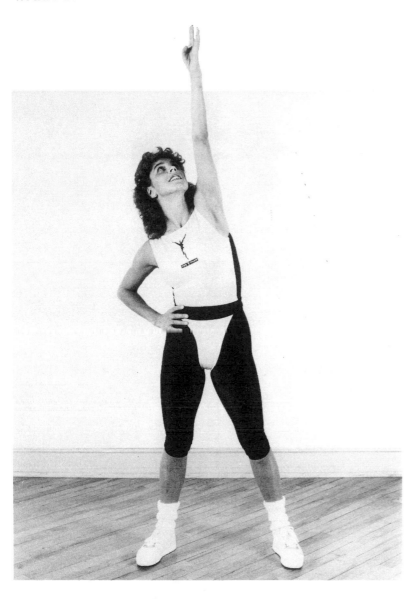

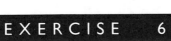

EXERCISE 6

Reaches

8

PURPOSE: TO GENERATE
HEAT, WARM THE
MUSCLES AND STRETCH
THE SIDES OF THE BODY

16

• Stand with feet shoulder-width apart, extend the right arm above the head and reach for the ceiling (1 count) then lower the arm down to the hip (1 count)

• Do this slowly 8 times, alternating right and left

Repeat

EXERCISE 3

Knee Bends and Arm Circles (p. 35)

8

16

Repeat

EXERCISE 4

Marches (p. 36)

16

16

Now go on to either the one-minute toning warm-up stretch overleaf or the one-minute aerobic warm-up stretch (p. 51), depending on which six-minute block you are doing.

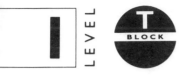

LEVEL T BLOCK

WARM - UP

Stretching (for muscle toning)

Breathe out as you go into stretches. Do not bounce in any position.

1

minute

EXERCISE 1

Standing Triceps Stretch

L + R

PURPOSE: TO STRETCH THE MUSCLE ALONG THE BACK OF THE UPPER ARM (TRICEPS)

16

• Stand with good posture and knees slightly bent, curve the left arm behind your head and place the fingers on the upper back between the shoulder blades

• Using the right hand, assist the stretch by gently pulling the left elbow across behind your head

• Hold for 8 counts then repeat for the right arm

> □ *Feel the stretch down the back of the upper arm*

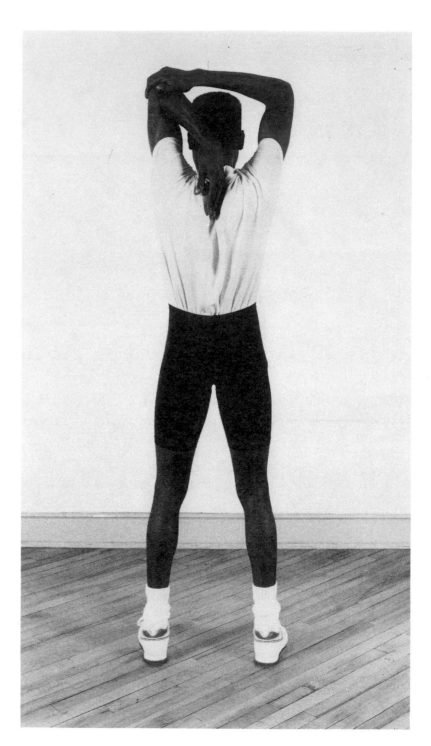

EXERCISE 2

Standing Shoulder Stretch

2

PURPOSE: TO STRETCH THE MUSCLES AROUND THE SHOULDERS

8

• Stand with good posture and knees slightly bent, clasp the hands together, pull in the stomach and extend the arms up above the head

• Try to pull the hands backwards to increase the stretch

• Hold for 4 counts, rest and repeat

□ *Feel the stretch around the shoulders*

□ *Maintain correct pelvic tilt*

□ *Don't arch the back*

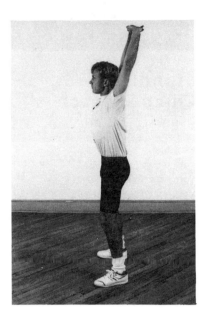

EXERCISE 3

Standing Chest Stretch

2

PURPOSE: TO STRETCH THE MUSCLES ACROSS THE FRONT OF THE CHEST (PECTORALS)

8

• Stand with good posture and knees slightly bent, clasping hands together behind the back

• Extend the arms out and up behind the back

• Hold for 4 counts, rest and repeat

□ *Feel the stretch across the front of the chest*

□ *Maintain correct pelvic tilt and don't bend forwards*

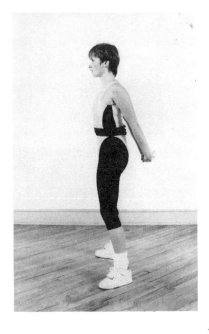

L E V E L **I**

T BLOCK

EXERCISE 4

Standing Quad Stretch

L + R

PURPOSE: TO STRETCH THE MUSCLES ALONG THE FRONT OF THE THIGH (QUADRICEPS)

16

- Face a wall or chair for support

- Transfer your weight to the right leg, bend the right knee slightly and tuck the buttocks under as for pelvic tilt

- Bring the left heel back and lift it up towards the buttocks, reaching for the left ankle with the left hand

- Use the left arm to bring the heel further up to increase the stretch

- Hold for 8 counts then repeat for the right leg

□ *Feel the stretch down the front of the thigh*

□ *Keep the back straight and the thighs parallel*

□ *Maintain correct pelvic tilt*

□ *If you don't feel a stretch, try to take the bent knee even further back.*

□ *If the bent knee is uncomfortable, try to extend the leg and the ankle will move slightly away from the body*

□ *If you can't reach the raised ankle, loop a towel round it and gradually pull the towel upwards*

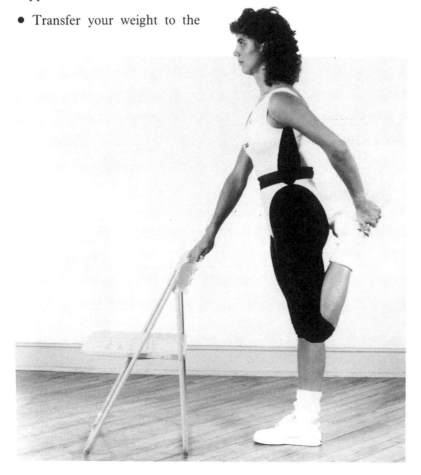

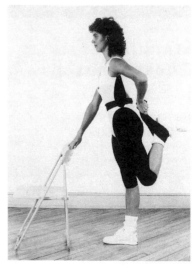

Now begin the muscle toning exercises opposite.

EXERCISES

(For muscle toning)

If at any time these exercises hurt, stop and check carefully that you are performing them correctly. If you think you are doing them correctly but you still feel uncomfortable, try the alternative exercises. All these exercises are new to you and your body, and it may take time to become familiar with the technique and/or for the body to adjust. Be patient. If necessary, miss out an exercise, go on to the next one and return to try again at a later date.

Think about and feel the particular muscle that is working. Control all movements and breathe out on effort. You will need a mat or something soft beneath you for this section.

6
minutes

EXERCISE 1

Pelvic Tilts
6

PURPOSE. TO STRENGTHEN THE STOMACH MUSCLES (ABDOMINALS)

24

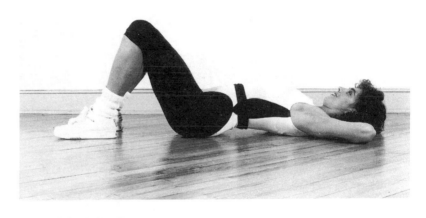

• Lie on your back, bend both knees, keeping them hip-distance apart, and place your hands on your stomach. Both feet should be flat on the floor

• Pull in your stomach and feel your lower back pushing into the floor. Lift your bottom slightly off the floor, against the downward pressure of your stomach muscles (2 counts)

• Relax for 2 counts

• Do this 6 times

☐ *Tilt your hips towards you*

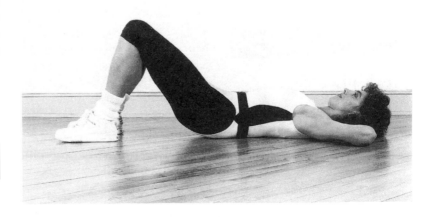

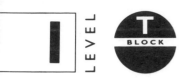

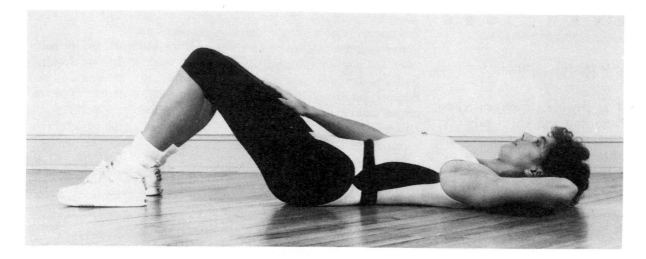

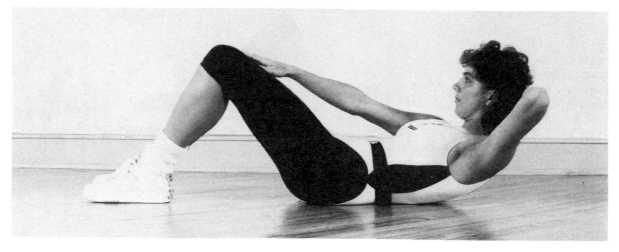

Either

EXERCISE   2A

Curl-Ups

8

PURPOSE: TO
STRENGTHEN THE
STOMACH MUSCLES
(ABDOMINALS)

32

• Lie on your back, both knees
bent and hip-distance apart, with
feet flat on the floor, your head
resting in the left hand and your
right hand on the right thigh

• Tilt your pelvis, feel the lower
back on the floor and curl up,
reaching your right hand over the
right knee, then relax (4 counts)

• Do this 8 times

☐ *Feel the stomach muscles
working and breathe out on
effort*

☐ *Keep the stomach pulled in
flat*

☐ *Keep knees bent and do not
pull on your head*

☐ *Tuck chin to chest*

LEVEL I

Or

EXERCISE 2B

Reverse Curl-Ups

8

PURPOSE: TO
STRENGTHEN THE
STOMACH MUSCLES
(ABDOMINALS)

32

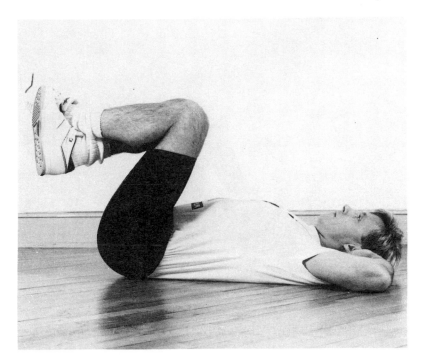

- Lie on your back, both knees bent up to the chest, and rest your head on both hands

- Tilt the pelvis and, keeping knees together, pull in with the stomach muscles to squeeze both knees towards your face. The buttocks and base of the spine will curl slowly off the floor (2 counts)

- Keeping stomach muscles pulled in, roll the base of the spine and buttocks back to the floor and relax (2 counts)

- Do this 8 times

□ *Feel the stomach muscles working*

□ *Keep the knees bent over the body at all times*

□ *Keep the movement smooth and slow*

□ *Place your arms by your sides with hands flat on the floor to help the movement*

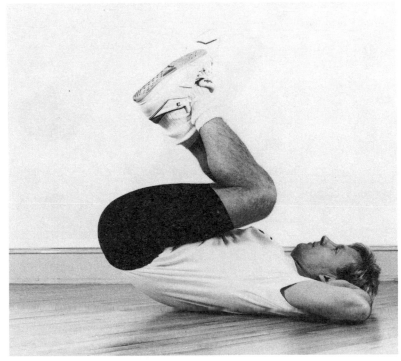

LEVEL **I**

T
BLOCK

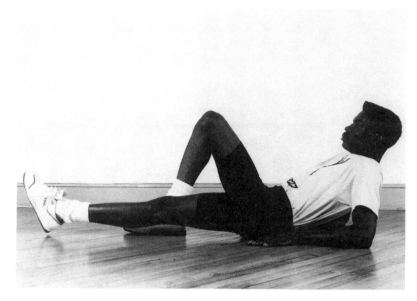

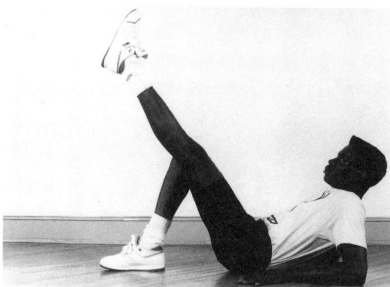

Either

EXERCISE 3A

Front Leg Raises

8L + 8R

PURPOSE: TO TONE UP
THE HIP FLEXORS AND
THE MUSCLES ALONG
THE FRONT OF THE
THIGH (QUADRICEPS)

16

• Lie on your back propped up on your elbows, one knee bent, one leg straight, hip-distance apart

• Tilt the pelvis, feeling the lower back pushing into the floor

• Raise your straight leg up to the height of the knee so that the thighs are parallel, then lower (1 count)

• Do this 8 times then repeat 8 times using the other leg

□ *Feel the thigh muscles working*

□ *Keep the working leg straight*

□ *Keep the stomach fixed and pulled in*

□ *Don't let the bottom or the back rock*

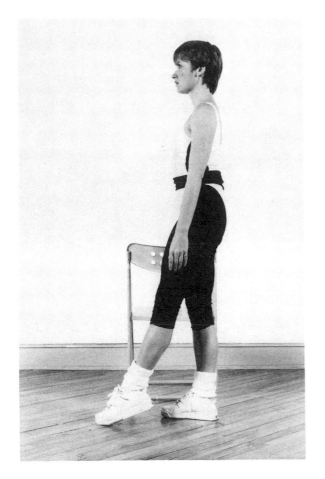

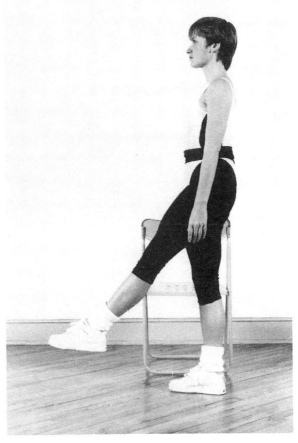

Or

EXERCISE 3B

Standing Front Leg Raises

8L + 8R

PURPOSE: TO TONE UP THE HIP FLEXORS AND THE MUSCLES ALONG THE FRONT OF THE THIGH (QUADRICEPS)

16

- Find a chair or wall for support and turn side-on to it

- Lean on the support with your right hand

- Lift your left leg, keeping it straight, approximately one foot off the ground, then lower (1 count)

- Do this 8 times then repeat 8 times using the right leg

□ *Feel the thigh muscles working*

□ *Keep good posture*

□ *Keep the working leg straight and don't lift it too high*

□ *Don't lift or lower it too quickly*

LEVEL

T BLOCK

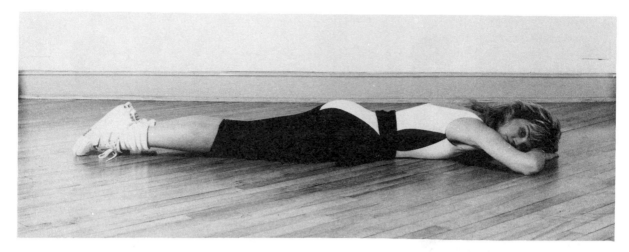

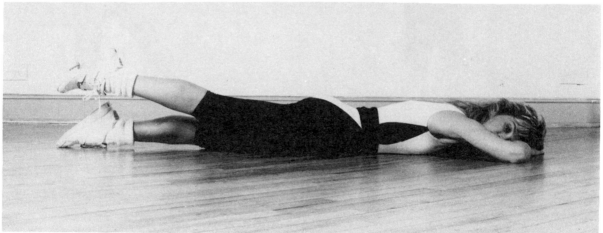

Either

EXERCISE 4A

Rear Leg Raises

8R + 8L

PURPOSE: TO TONE THE MUSCLES IN THE BACK OF THE THIGH (HAMSTRINGS) AND BUTTOCKS (GLUTEALS)

16

- Lie on your stomach, legs straight out behind. Place your hands flat on the floor under your face

- Keeping both hips pressed into the floor, raise your right leg, then lower (1 count)

- Do this 8 times then repeat 8 times using the left leg

☐ *Feel the muscles at the back of your thigh working*

☐ *The leg will not go very high*

☐ *Keep the legs straight*

☐ *If the back hurts, try the next exercise as an alternative*

Or

EXERCISE 4B

Standing Rear Leg Raises

8L + 8R

PURPOSE: TO TONE THE MUSCLES IN THE BACK OF THE THIGH (HAMSTRINGS) AND BUTTOCKS (GLUTEALS)

16

- Stand facing a chair, leaning slightly forwards to use its support and place the left leg straight out behind

- Lift and lower the left leg, keeping the stomach tight and the back straight (1 count)

- Do this 8 times then repeat 8 times using the right leg

☐ *Feel the muscle at the back of your thigh working*

☐ *If the back hurts, don't lift the leg so high*

☐ *Keep the stomach tight*

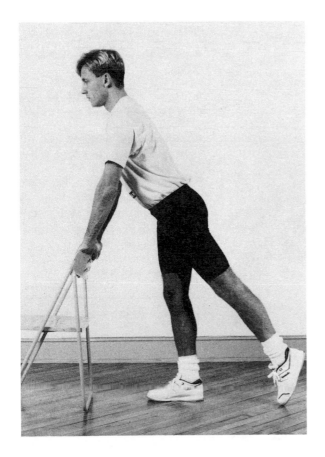

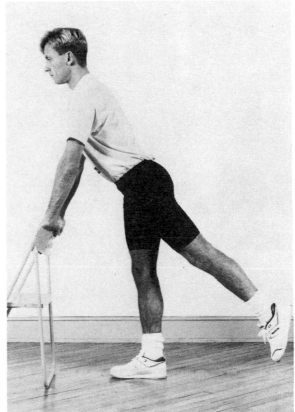

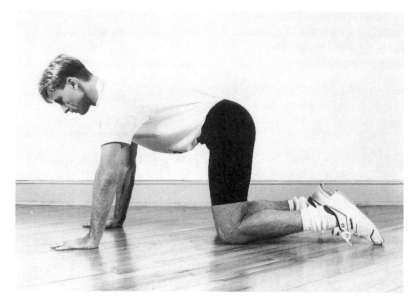

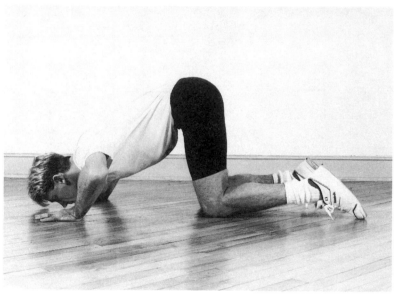

Either

EXERCISE 5A

Box Press-Ups
8

PURPOSE: TO
STRENGTHEN THE
MUSCLES IN THE BACK
OF THE UPPER ARMS
(TRICEPS) AND CHEST
(PECTORALS)

16

- Come up on to all fours and place your hands with fingers facing forward shoulder-width apart

- Place the shoulders over your hands

- Make sure your hips are directly above your knees

- Pull in your stomach and tilt your pelvis until your back is flat

- Bend your elbows, lowering your forehead to the floor (1 count), then push up, straightening the elbows, but don't snap them! (1 count)

- Do this 8 times

□ *Feel the arms working*

□ *Constantly check your position*

□ *Don't round the shoulders*

□ *Breathe regularly*

LEVEL I

Or

EXERCISE 5B

Standing Press-Ups

8

PURPOSE: TO
STRENGTHEN THE
MUSCLES IN THE BACK
OF THE UPPER ARMS
(TRICEPS) AND CHEST
(PECTORALS)

16

• Stand approximately one foot away from the wall, feet shoulder-width apart and hands touching the wall slightly more than shoulder-width apart, in line with the head

• Slowly bend the elbows, lowering the body weight towards the wall (1 count), then slowly straighten the arms to push the body away from the wall (1 count)

• Do this 8 times

☐ *Feel the arms working*

☐ *Don't snap the elbows, extend them smoothly*

☐ *Keep the back and body straight*

☐ *Keep the stomach muscles tight*

☐ *Breathe normally*

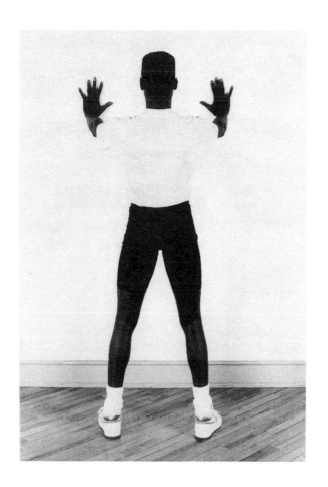 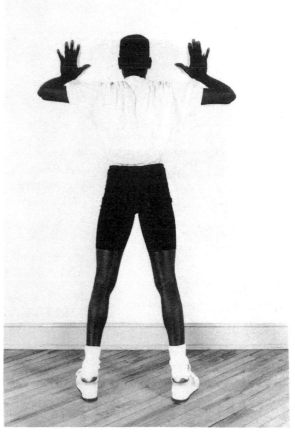

LEVEL

T BLOCK

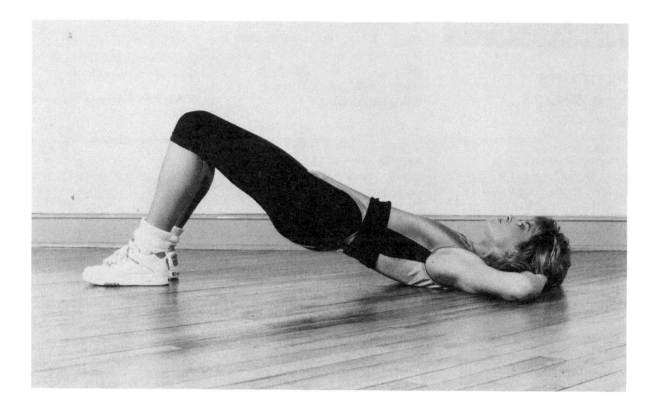

EXERCISE   6

Buttock Squeezes

8

PURPOSE: TO TONE UP
THE BUTTOCK MUSCLES
(GLUTEALS)

16

- Lay on your back, flatten the stomach, and tilt the hips towards you as in the pelvic tilt

- Lift the hips slightly further off the floor

- Squeeze the buttocks keeping the lower back still, then relax the buttocks, keeping the hips still (2 counts)

- Do this 8 times

☐ *Feel the buttocks working*

☐ *Take care to keep the upper back (shoulder blades) in contact with the floor*

☐ *Keep the movement smooth and controlled without jerking*

☐ *Breathe normally throughout*

Repeat

EXERCISES   1–6

two more times. This should take 6 minutes in all.

Now go on to Level 1 cool-down (p. 58).

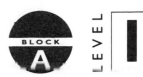

WARM - UP

....

Stretching (for aerobics)

Breathe out as you go into stretches. Do not bounce in any position.

|

minute

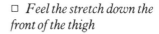

EXERCISE 1

Standing Quad Stretch

L + R

PURPOSE: TO STRETCH THE MUSCLES ALONG THE FRONT OF THE THIGH (QUADRICEPS)

16

....

• Face a wall or chair for support

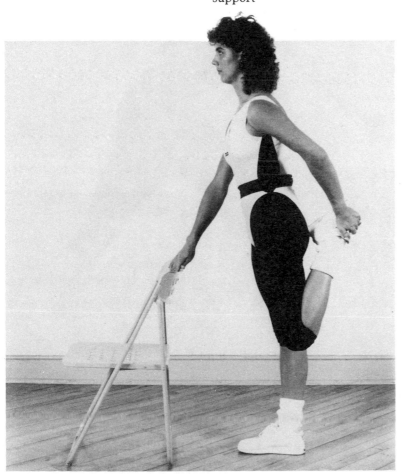

• Transfer your weight to the right leg, bend the right knee slightly and tuck the bottom under as for pelvic tilt

• Bring the left heel back and up towards the buttocks, reaching for the left ankle with the left hand

• Use the left arm to bring the heel further up to increase the stretch

• Hold for 8 counts then repeat for the right leg

□ *Feel the stretch down the front of the thigh*

□ *Keep the back straight and the thighs parallel*

□ *Maintain correct pelvic tilt*

□ *If you don't feel a stretch, try to take the bent knee even further back*

□ *If the bent knee is uncomfortable, try to extend the leg and the ankle will move slightly away from the body*

□ *If you can't reach the raised ankle, loop a towel round it and gradually pull the towel upwards*

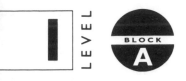

EXERCISE 2

Standing Calf Stretch

L + R

PURPOSE: TO STRETCH
THE MUSCLE ALONG THE
BACK OF THE LOWER LEG
(GASTROCNEMIUS)

16

• Stand with feet shoulder-width apart, three feet from a wall or chair for support, then step forward on to the right foot, bending the knee to take most of your weight, leaning on your support for balance

• Keep the left leg straight and push the heel flat to the floor

• Hold for 8 counts then repeat for the right leg

□ *Feel the stretch down the back of the lower leg*

□ *Check that both feet are facing forwards*

□ *If the stretch is too strong, take the front leg back and put less weight on it*

□ *Check that your feet stay shoulder-width apart to aid balance*

□ *Squeeze the buttocks to stabilise the hips*

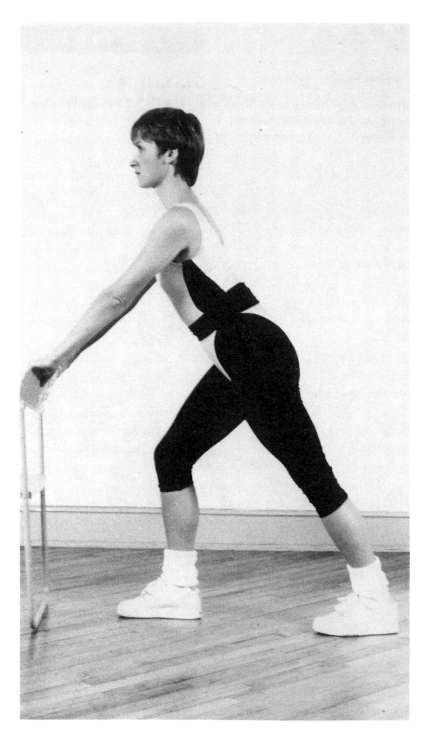

BLOCK
A

LEVEL
I

EXERCISE 3

Standing Lower Calf Stretch

L + R

PURPOSE: TO STRETCH
THE MUSCLE ALONG THE
BACK OF THE LOWER LEG
(SOLEUS) AND THE BACK
OF THE ANKLE
(ACHILLES TENDON)

16

- Assume the same position as for the Standing Calf Stretch

- Bring the back leg forwards a little

- Squeezing the buttocks, tilt the pelvis correctly to stabilise the hips, then bend the back leg and press the heel into the floor

- Hold for 8 counts then repeat for the right leg

□ *Feel the stretch lower down the calf of the back leg*

□ *Check that the back foot faces forwards and knee is in line with toe*

□ *Squeeze the buttocks to stabilise the hips*

□ *If you have difficulty with balance, check that your feet are not behind one another but shoulder-width apart*

□ *Remember to take most of your weight on the back leg*

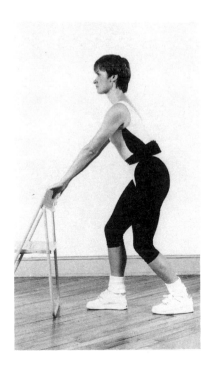

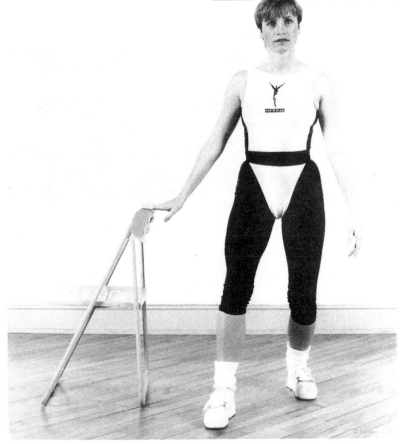

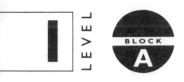

LEVEL I

BLOCK A

EXERCISE 4

Standing Shoulder Stretch

2

PURPOSE: TO STRETCH
THE MUSCLES AROUND
THE SHOULDERS

8

• Stand with good posture and knees slightly bent, clasp the hands together, pull in the stomach and extend the arms up above the head

• Try to pull the hands backwards to increase the stretch

• Hold for 4 counts, rest and repeat

> ☐ *Feel the stretch around the shoulders*
>
> ☐ *Maintain correct pelvic tilt*
>
> ☐ *Don't arch the back*

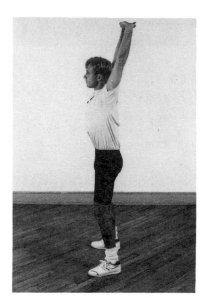

EXERCISE 5

Standing Chest Stretch

2

PURPOSE: TO STRETCH
THE MUSCLES ACROSS
THE FRONT OF THE
CHEST (PECTORALS)

8

• Stand with good posture and knees slightly bent, clasp the hands together behind the back

• Extend the arms out and up behind the back

• Hold for 4 counts, rest and repeat

> ☐ *Feel the stretch across the front of the chest*
>
> ☐ *Maintain correct pelvic tilt and don't bend forwards*

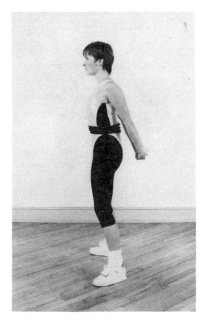

Now begin the aerobic exercises opposite.

EXERCISES

(For aerobics)

Make sure that you start slowly with these exercises and take your time to work faster. All of these exercises are designed to work the large muscle groups, heart and lungs. You should feel quite warm when you do these exercises.

The aerobic exercises should be done in continuous sequences. What follows are the instructions for the individual exercises and the order in which they should be performed.

If an exercise feels uncomfortable or too difficult, make the movements slower and/or don't use your arms and/or make the steps smaller, but keep the sequence continuous. When jogging or jumping you can make the exercise easier by keeping one foot or both feet in contact with the ground. Always remember to bend the knees, ankles and feet slightly on landing or making contact with the floor.

Breathe normally. If you become very breathless, make the exercises easier as suggested above. If you get tired, don't stop but walk on the spot until you can continue with the exercises again or until the six minutes are up.

6
minutes

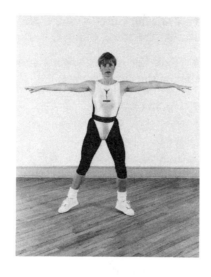

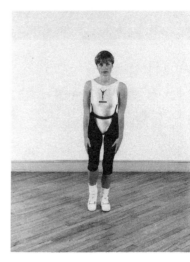

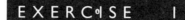

EXERCISE 1

Step Tap + Step Tap with Arms
8 + 8 **32**

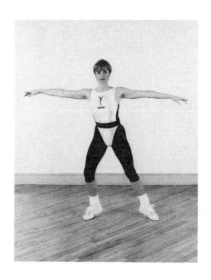

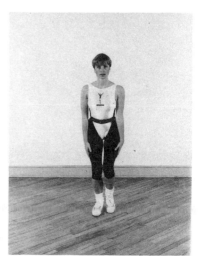

- Step sideways on to the right foot, tap the left foot next to it with a little knee bend (1 count), then repeat to the left (1 count)

- Do the full exercise 8 times

- Repeat 8 times more, lifting the arms out to the sides on the step and slapping the thighs on the tap

LEVEL I

BLOCK A

EXERCISE 2

Walks

4 Fwds + Bwds and
4 L + R   **32**

- Walk forwards 4 steps and clap on the 4th (2 counts)

- Walk backwards 4 steps and clap on the 4th (2 counts)

- Do this 4 times

- Walk to the right for 4 steps and clap on the 4th (2 counts)

- Walk to the left for 4 steps and clap on the 4th (2 counts)

- Do this 4 times

EXERCISE 3

Twists and Marches

(8 + 8) × 2   **32**

- Stand with feet hip-width apart, putting your weight on the balls of your feet

- Jump and twist shoulders to face diagonally left, and feet and knees to face diagonally right (1 count)

- Do this 8 times alternating right and left

- March on the spot, right and left, lifting the knees high with

each step and swinging your bent arms vigorously (1 count)

- Do this 8 times then repeat both exercises

☐ *Swivel on your toes if you don't want to jump in the twists*

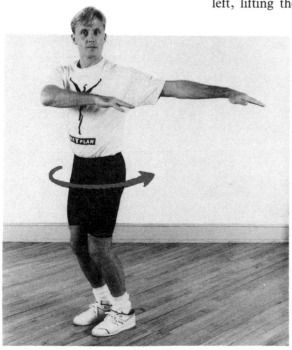

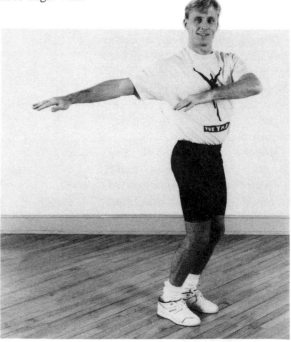

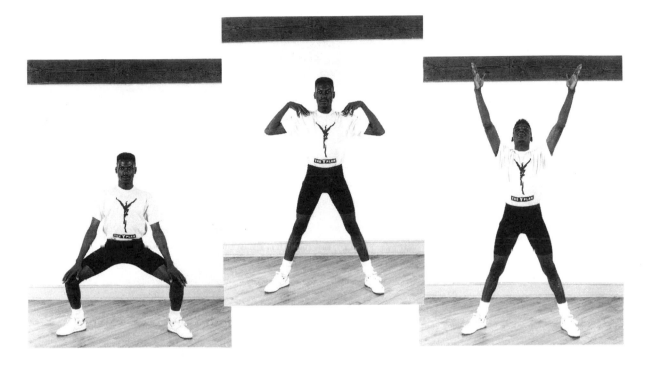

EXERCISE 4

Squat and Reach

| 2   **24**

● Stand with feet wider than shoulder-width apart, clap once then bend the knees as far as possible, keeping the heels pressed down, the knees out over the toes and the hips higher than the knees (1 count)

● Stand upright, tapping the hands to the shoulders as you do so then reaching both arms to the ceiling (1 count)

● Do this 12 times

> □ *Keep the back straight and upright with feet flat on the floor*
>
> □ *Push the knees out over the toes*
>
> □ *Don't let the buttocks go lower than the knees*
>
> □ *If the exercise is too difficult, don't bend the knees so far*

Repeat

EXERCISES 1–4

two more times. This should take 6 minutes in all.

Take it gently at first to give your body time to adjust. Work hard the second time, then take it easy again the third time to allow your body the chance to cool down gradually.

If you get through the whole exercise sequence in less than 6 minutes, next time do your second sequence once or twice more.

Now go on to Level 1 cool-down overleaf.

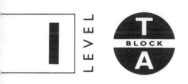

COOL-DOWN

Stretching (for muscle toning and aerobics)

Have something comfortable and cushioning beneath you, like a towel or carpet. Breathe out as you go into a stretch and try to relax in all stretched positions. If the stretches are uncomfortable, do not hold them for so long. If you feel a longer cool-down would be helpful, repeat the warm-up mobility and pulse-raising exercises on p. 33 after this stretching section, but keep the movements slow and relaxed.

3

minutes

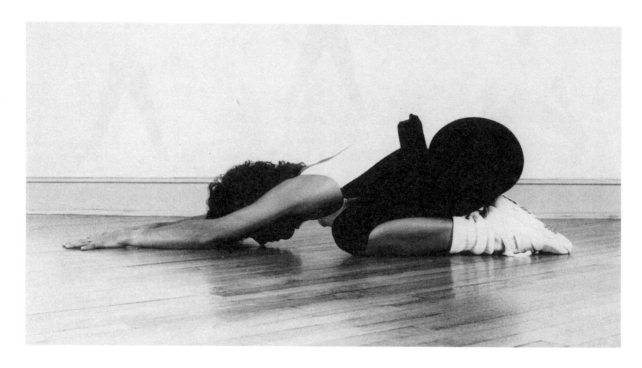

EXERCISE 1

Kneeling Shoulder Stretch

PURPOSE: TO STRETCH THE MUSCLES AROUND THE SHOULDERS

16

• Kneeling, sit back on your heels then lean forwards so that the chest rests on the thighs

• Stretch the arms straight forwards and place your hands on the floor in front of you, thumbs close together

• Push your chest towards the floor and hold for 16 counts

☐ *Feel the stretch around your shoulders*

☐ *Keep your stomach tight to prevent the back from arching*

☐ *Look down at the floor*

☐ *To increase the stretch, separate your knees and push your chest down between them*

58

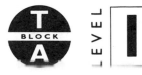

EXERCISE 2

Lying Stomach Stretch

2

PURPOSE: TO STRETCH
THE STOMACH MUSCLES
(ABDOMINALS) AND TO
MOBILISE THE SPINE

16

• Lie on your front and place your hands flat on the floor in front of your head, with arms slightly bent

• Gently lift the head and shoulders off the floor by pushing on your hands and straightening your arms. Keeping your hips on the floor, walk your hands back towards you until you feel a stretch down your stomach

• Hold for 8 counts, rest and repeat

☐ *Look ahead and keep your hip bones on the floor*

☐ *If your back aches, lower your shoulders further or leave this exercise out*

☐ *Think of lengthening your spine*

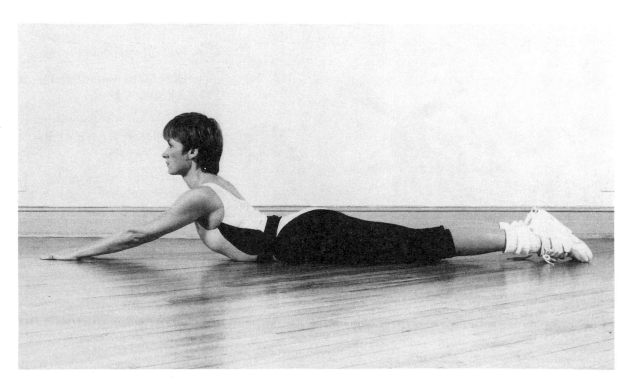

LEVEL I

BLOCK T A

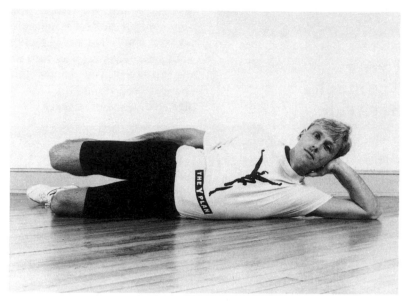

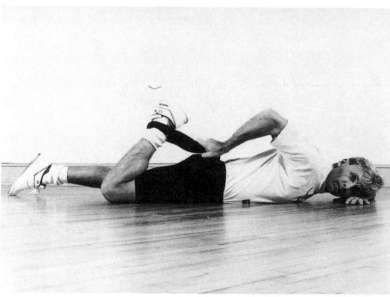

EXERCISE 3

Side-Lying Quad Stretch

L + R

PURPOSE: TO STRETCH
OUT THE MUSCLES
ALONG THE FRONT OF
THE THIGH
(QUADRICEPS)

32

- Lie on your right side with the body straight and with knees bent at right-angles to the body. Rest your head in your right hand

- Bend the left leg, hold the left ankle with the left hand and gently pull it back towards your buttocks

- Feel the stretch in the thigh

- Hold for 16 counts then repeat on the other side

□ *Take care not to twist or hollow the back*

□ *Keep the underneath leg bent for stability*

□ *Don't pull too hard on the ankle*

□ *If the stretch is too much, loop a towel round the ankle or roll on to your front and wrap a towel round your foot, using it to assist your stretch*

E X E R C I S E   4

Sitting Groin Stretch

PURPOSE: TO STRETCH
THE MUSCLES OF THE
INNER THIGH
(ADDUCTORS)

32

• Sit on the floor and bring the soles of the feet together as close to the groin as possible

• Place a hand on each ankle and press the knees towards the floor with the elbows until you feel a stretch in the groin

• Hold for 32 counts, trying to relax the muscles. If you feel the stretch becomes easier, press down with the elbows a little more to develop the stretch and improve your flexibility

☐ *Sit up as straight as possible*

☐ *Keep the shoulders down*

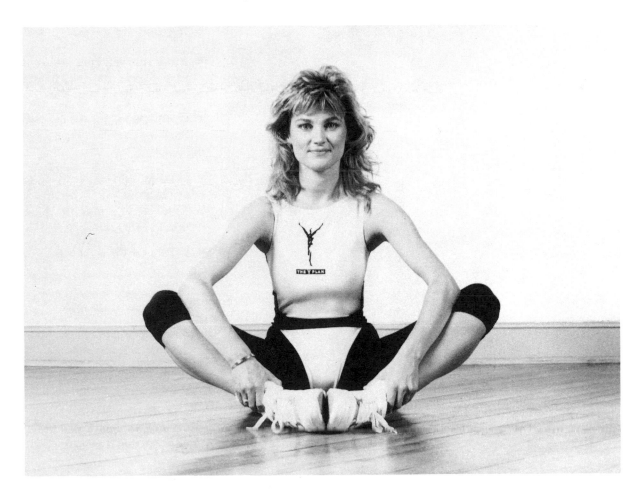

LEVEL **1**

T
BLOCK
A

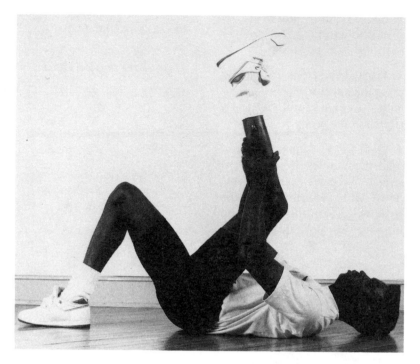

EXERCISE 5

Lying Hamstring Stretch

L + R

PURPOSE: TO STRETCH
THE MUSCLES AT THE
BACK OF THE LEG
(HAMSTRINGS)

32

- Lie on your back with both knees bent and both feet flat on the floor

- Bring your left knee into your chest and hold the calf, fingers below, thumbs on your shin

- Gently extend the left leg until you feel the stretch in the back of the thigh

- Hold for 16 counts, trying to relax the muscles. If the stretch becomes easier, pull the knee further towards the chest

- Repeat for the right leg

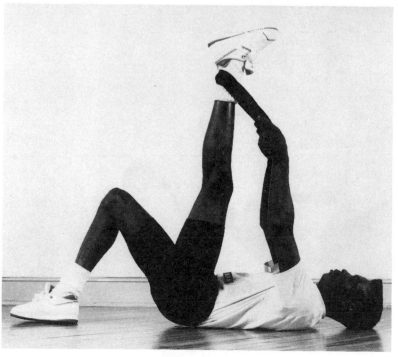

□ *Keep head, shoulders and base of spine on the floor*

□ *Keep your hips square so as not to twist the back*

□ *The leg being stretched does not need to straighten*

□ *If this is uncomfortable, loop a towel round your ankle and pull it gently towards you*

BLOCK T A

LEVEL 1

EXERCISE 6

Standing Calf Stretch

L + R

PURPOSE: TO STRETCH THE MUSCLE ALONG THE BACK OF THE LOWER LEG (GASTROCNEMIUS)

16

• Stand with feet shoulder-width apart about three feet from a wall or chair for support, then step forward on to the right foot, bending the knee to take most of your weight, leaning on your support for balance

• Keep the left leg straight and push the heel flat to the floor

• Hold for 8 counts then repeat for the right leg

□ *Feel the stretch down the back of the lower leg*

□ *Check that both feet are facing forwards.*

□ *Check that your feet stay shoulder-width apart to aid balance*

□ *Squeeze the buttocks to stabilise the hips*

□ *If the stretch is too strong, take the front leg back and put less weight on it*

EXERCISE 7

Standing Lower Calf Stretch

L + R

PURPOSE: TO STRETCH THE MUSCLE ALONG THE BACK OF THE LOWER LEG (SOLEUS) AND THE BACK OF THE ANKLE (ACHILLES TENDON)

16

• Assume the same position as for the Standing Calf Stretch

• Bring the back leg forwards a little

• Squeezing the buttocks, tilt

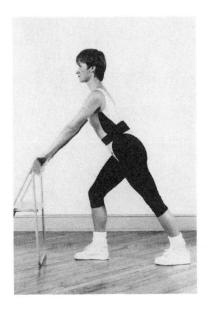

---

the pelvis correctly to stabilise the hips, then bend the back leg and press the heel into the floor

• Hold for 8 counts then repeat for the right leg

□ *Feel the stretch lower down the calf of the back leg*

□ *Check that the back foot faces forwards and knee is in line with toe*

□ *Squeeze the buttocks to stabilise the hips*

□ *If you have difficulty with balance, check that your feet are not behind one another but shoulder-width apart*

□ *Remember to take most of your weight on the back leg*

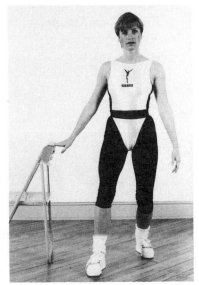

I

L E V E L

T
BLOCK
A

EXERCISE 8

Standing Triceps Stretch

L + R

PURPOSE: TO STRETCH
THE MUSCLE ALONG THE
BACK OF THE UPPER ARM
(TRICEPS)

16

- Stand with good posture and knees slightly bent, curve the left arm behind the head and place the fingers on the upper back between the shoulder blades

- Using the right hand, assist the stretch by gently pulling the left elbow across behind the head

- Hold for 8 counts then repeat for the right arm

> □ *Feel the stretch down the back of the upper arm*

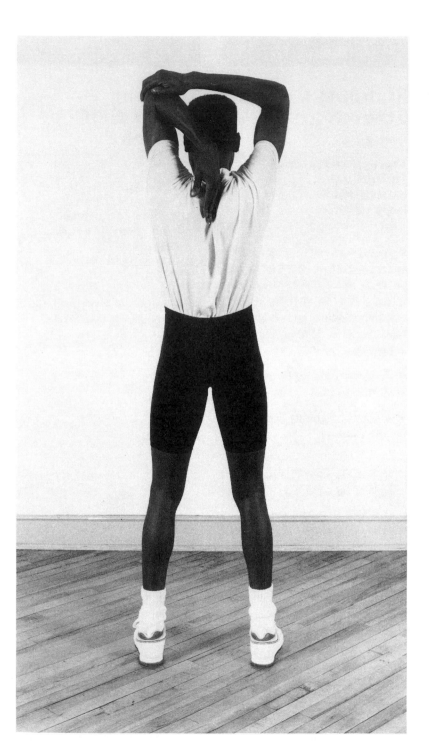

W A R M - U P

The warm-up section is divided into two parts.

The first two minutes are always done regardless of whether your main exercise block on a given day is for toning or aerobics.

You then follow this with one minute of stretching for either the toning warm-up or the aerobic warm-up. After completing the appropriate warm-up, you go on to six minutes of toning or aerobic exercise, followed by the three-minute cool-down.

Mobility and pulse-raising (for muscle toning and aerobics)

Always check posture and work through the full range of movement. Exercise to generate heat and warm the muscles. Remember to count 'one and' for one second.

2
minutes

E X E R C I S E   1

Heel and Toe with Arm Extensions

8R + 8L

PURPOSE: TO MOBILISE THE ANKLE

16

● Stand with all your weight on the left leg with the left knee slightly bent

● With the right foot, tap heel and toe on the floor, at the same

time pushing the arms forwards from the chest with the heel tap and pulling them in again with each toe tap (heel + toe = 1 count)

● Do this 8 times then repeat with the left foot

□ *Feel the movement in the ankle*

□ *Keep the hips level*

□ *The knee of the supporting leg should be over the toe*

□ *Flex and point the working toe as far as possible*

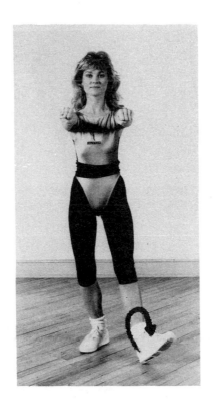

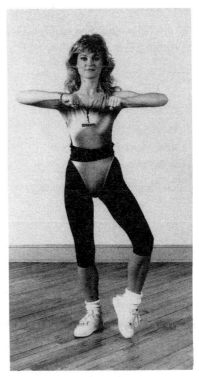

2 LEVEL

T
BLOCK
A

EXERCISE 2

Side Bends

4R + 4L

PURPOSE: TO MOBILISE
THE SPINE AND STRETCH
THE SIDES OF THE BODY

16

- Stand with feet shoulder-width apart, knees slightly bent and with correct pelvic tilt

- Lean the upper body over to the right over the right hip, sliding the right hand down towards the outside of the right knee and at the same time sliding the left hand up under the left armpit, then return to centre (2 counts)

- Do this 8 times, alternating right and left

□ *Feel a slight stretch in your side*

□ *Keep the body straight; don't lean backwards or forwards*

□ *Keep your weight evenly over both feet*

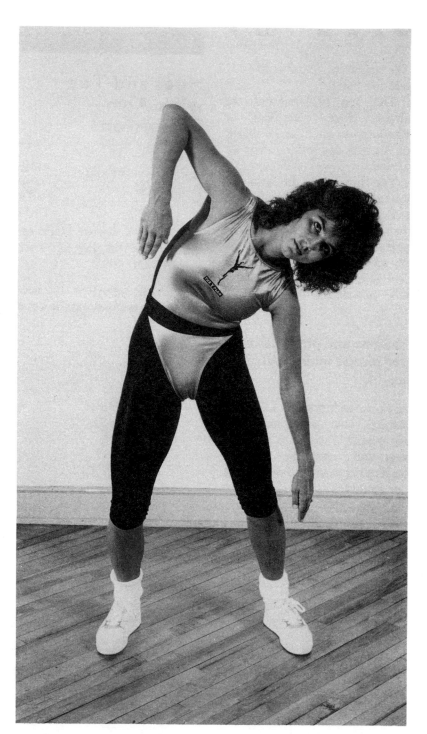

T
BLOCK
A

LEVEL
2

EXERCISE   3

Squat and Reach

8

PURPOSE: TO GENERATE
HEAT AND WARM THE
MUSCLES

16

- Stand with feet wider than shoulder-width apart, clap once then bend the knees as far as possible, keeping the heels pressed down, the knees out over the toes and the hips higher than the knees (1 count)

- Stand upright, tapping the hands to the shoulders as you do so and reaching both arms high to the ceiling (1 count)

- Do this 8 times

☐ *Keep the back straight and upright with feet flat on the floor*

☐ *Push the knees out over the toes*

☐ *Don't let the buttocks go lower than the knees*

☐ *If the exercise is too difficult, don't bend the knees so far*

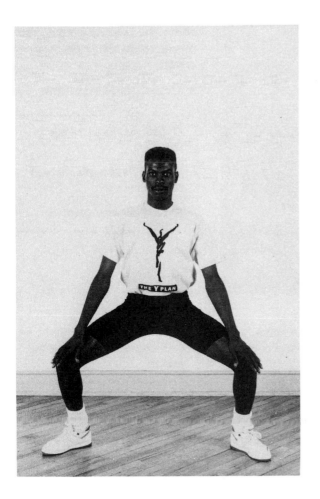

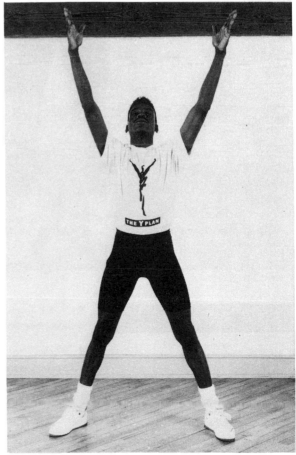

2 LEVEL T BLOCK A

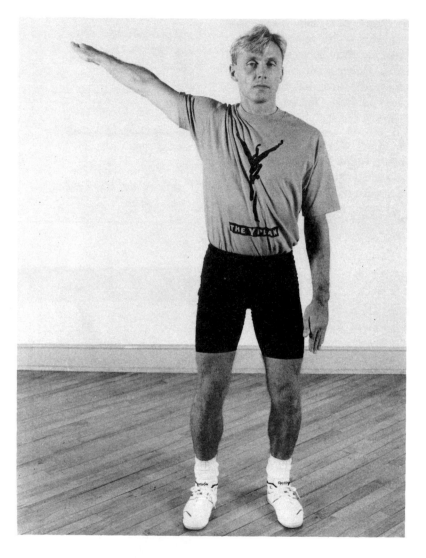

EXERCISE 4

Arm Circles
4

PURPOSE: TO MOBILISE THE SHOULDERS

8

- Stand with feet shoulder-width apart, knees slightly bent, keeping the buttocks and stomach tight

- Circle the left arm backwards above the head (2 counts) then repeat with the right arm (2 counts)

- Repeat once for each arm

> □ *Feel the movement in your shoulder*
>
> □ *Take the straight arm back past your ear*
>
> □ *Keep the hips square-on*

EXERCISE 5

Walks
4

PURPOSE: TO GENERATE HEAT AND WARM THE MUSCLES

16

- Walk forwards 4 steps, clap hands once on the 4th (2 counts)

- Walk backwards 4 steps, clapping once on the 4th (2 counts)

- Do this 4 times

> □ *Swing arms throughout the walks*

EXERCISE 6

Hip Circles
4R + 4L

PURPOSE: TO MOBILISE
THE LOWER BACK

16

• Stand with feet shoulder-width apart and knees slightly bent

• Circle the hips by taking them to the right, backwards, to the left, then forwards, using the stomach muscles (2 counts)

• Do this 4 times to the right and 4 to the left

> ☐ *Feel your stomach muscles assisting the movement*
>
> ☐ *Keep your knees slightly flexed and over your feet*
>
> ☐ *Keep the shoulders still*

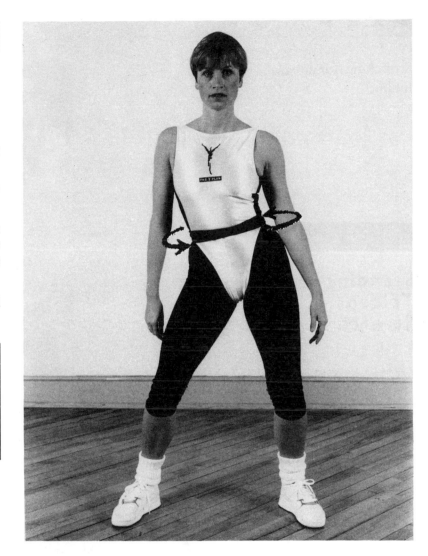

Repeat

EXERCISE 3

Squat and Reach (p. 67)

8

16

Repeat

EXERCISE 5

Walks (p. 68)

4

16

Now go on to either the one-minute toning warm-up stretch overleaf or the one-minute aerobic warm-up stretch on p. 82, depending on which six-minute block you are doing.

WARM-UP

Stretching (for muscle toning)

|

minute

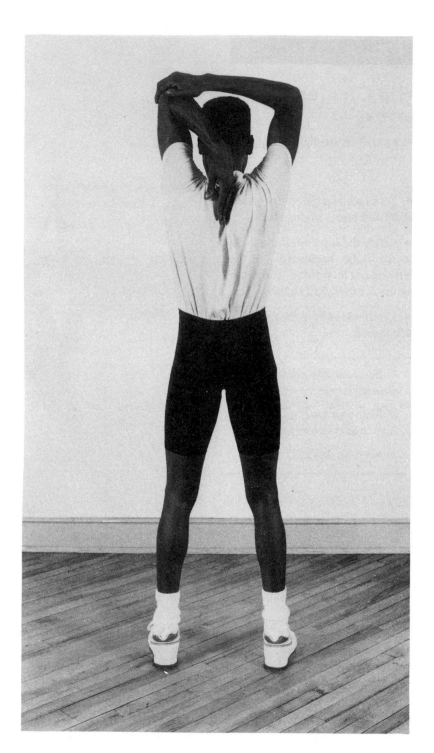

EXERCISE 1

Standing Triceps Stretch

L + R

PURPOSE: TO STRETCH THE MUSCLE ALONG THE BACK OF THE UPPER ARM (TRICEPS)

16

- Stand with good posture and knees slightly bent, curve the left arm back over the head and place the fingers on the upper back between the shoulder blades

- Using the right hand, assist the stretch by gently pulling the left elbow across behind the head

- Hold for 8 counts then repeat for the right arm

☐ *Feel the stretch down the back of the upper arm*

EXERCISE 2

Sitting Hamstring Stretch

L + R

PURPOSE: TO STRETCH
THE MUSCLES AT THE
BACK OF THE THIGH
(HAMSTRINGS)

16

● Sit on the floor, with left leg straight out in front and right leg slightly to the side, bent out of way

● Sit up tall and place your hands on the floor either side of your left leg

● Pull in the stomach and, trying to keep your back straight, bend forwards over the straight leg until you feel the stretch down the back of the left leg.

● Hold for 8 counts, then slowly come out of the stretch and repeat for the right leg

□ *Keep the hips square*

□ *Be content not to reach your nose to your shin!*

□ *If you feel a pull in your back, try the Lying Hamstring Stretch from cool-down in Level 1 (see p. 62)*

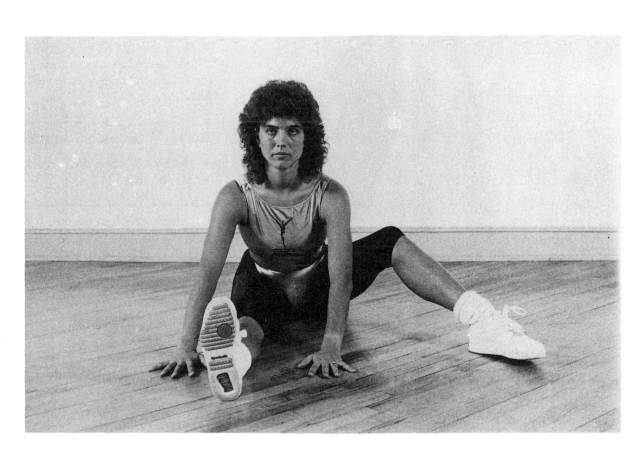

2 LEVEL

T BLOCK

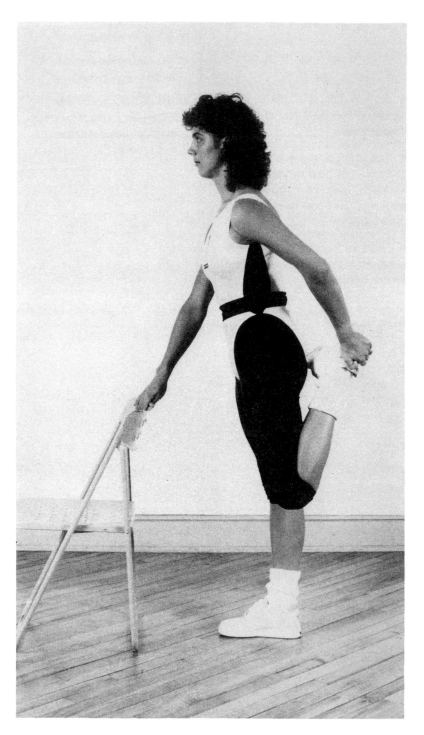

EXERCISE 3

Standing Quad Stretch

L + R

PURPOSE: TO STRETCH THE MUSCLES ALONG THE FRONT OF THE THIGH (QUADRICEPS)

16

- Face a wall or chair for support

- Transfer your weight to the right leg, bend the right knee slightly and tuck the buttocks under as for pelvic tilt

- Bring the left heel back and lift it up towards the buttocks, reaching for the left ankle with the left hand

- Use the left arm to bring the heel up to increase the stretch

- Hold for 8 counts then repeat for the right leg

□ *Feel the stretch down the front of the thigh*

□ *Keep the back straight and the thighs parallel*

□ *If you don't feel a stretch, try to take the bent knee even further back*

□ *If the bent knee is uncomfortable, try to extend the leg and the ankle will move slightly away from the body*

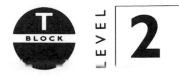

EXERCISE 4

Standing Shoulder Stretch

2

PURPOSE: TO STRETCH
THE MUSCLES AROUND
THE SHOULDERS

8

- Stand with good posture and knees slightly bent, clasp the hands together, pull in the stomach and extend the arms up above the head

- Try to pull the hands backwards to increase the stretch

- Hold for 4 counts, rest and repeat

> □ *Feel the stretch around the shoulders*
>
> □ *Maintain correct pelvic tilt*
>
> □ *Don't arch the back*

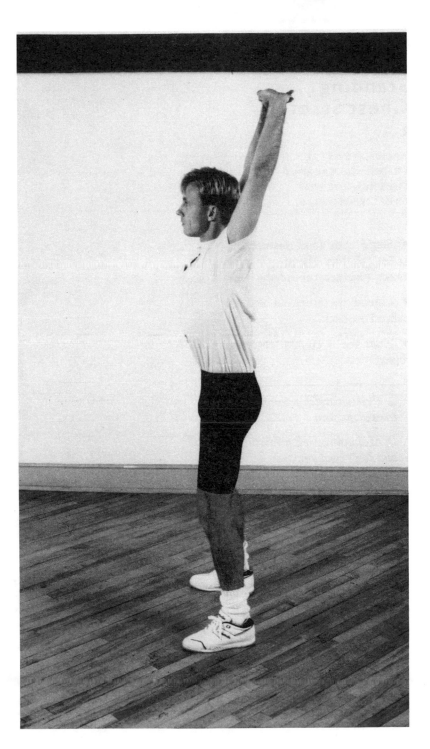

2 L E V E L

T **BLOCK**

E X E R C I S E 5

Standing Chest Stretch
2

PURPOSE: TO STRETCH THE MUSCLES ACROSS THE FRONT OF THE CHEST (PECTORALS)

8

- Stand with good posture and knees slightly bent, clasping hands together behind the back

- Extend the arms out and up behind the back

- Hold for 4 counts, rest and repeat

☐ *Feel the stretch across the front of the chest*

☐ *Maintain correct pelvic tilt and don't bend forwards*

Now begin the muscle toning exercises opposite.

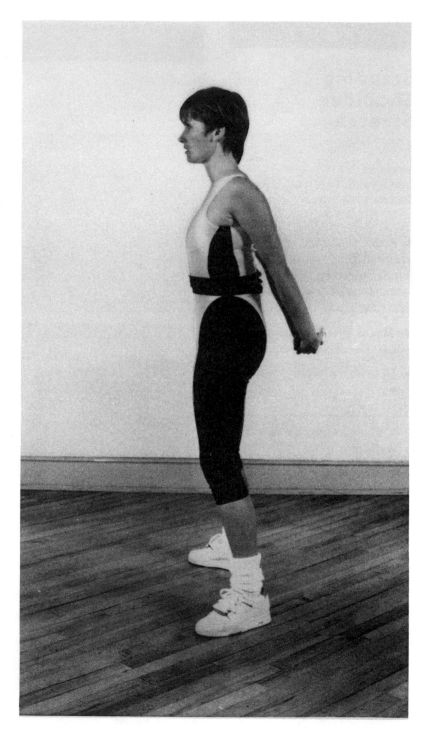

EXERCISES

(For muscle toning)

Breathe out with the effort of every exercise and make the fullest range of movement possible for each exercise. Move with control and check your exercise technique continually. You will need a chair or a wall for support in Exercises 1–3.

6

minutes

EXERCISE 1

Standing Side Leg Raises

6R × 2

PURPOSE: TO STRENGTHEN THE MUSCLES ON THE OUTSIDE OF THE THIGH (ABDUCTORS)

32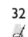

● Stand left-side-on to a wall or chair for support, with your weight on the left leg

● Place your right toes on the floor, slightly behind but squeezing both thighs together

● Keeping the right leg slightly bent, raise the right leg out to side (1 count), keeping your hips still and your right knee facing forwards. Relax (1 count)

● Do this 6 times (12 counts), rest for 8 counts then repeat the exercise 6 more times, still on the right leg (12 counts)

☐ *Feel your outside thigh muscles working*

☐ *Keep the body square and your hips level*

☐ *You may prefer to bend the supporting leg slightly*

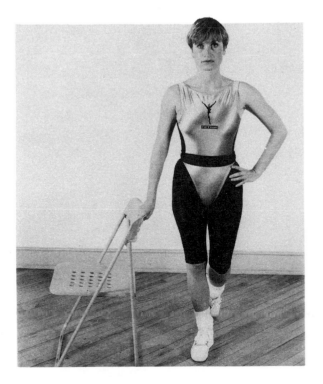

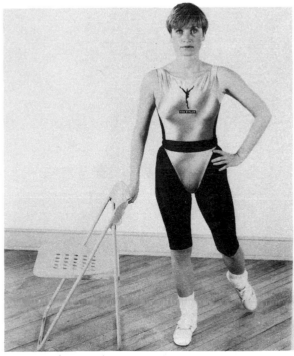

2

LEVEL

T BLOCK

EXERCISE 2

Forward Squats

4 L

PURPOSE: TO
STRENGTHEN THE THIGH
MUSCLES (QUADRICEPS
AND HAMSTRINGS) AND
THE BUTTOCK MUSCLES
(GLUTEALS)

16

• Stand with feet hip-width apart, right-side-on to a wall or chair for support, using it for balance with your hand.

• Stride forward with the left foot so that the back right heel comes off the floor, with your weight on the right toes and left foot, then bend the knees, keeping the back upright, until the back knee almost touches the floor near but behind your left heel (2 counts)

• Straighten the legs (2 counts)

• Do this complete exercise 4 times

☐ *Feel your thighs working as you use the strength of the thighs to lift you up at the back*

☐ *Squeeze the buttocks tight to support the hips*

☐ *Only go down as far as is comfortable; don't worry if at first you don't reach the floor*

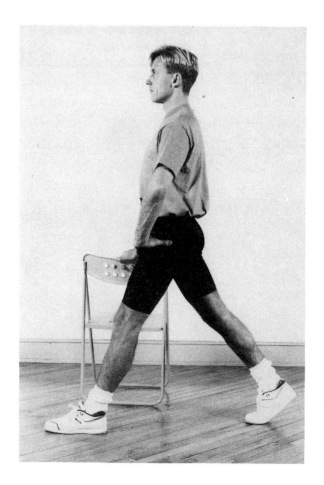

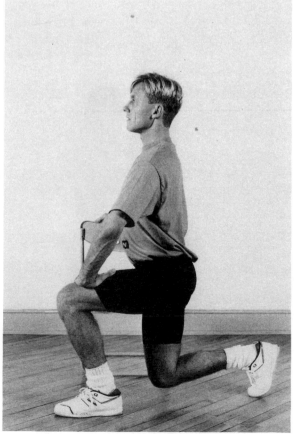

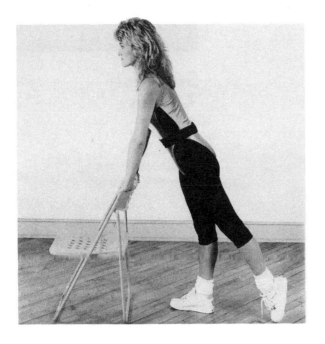
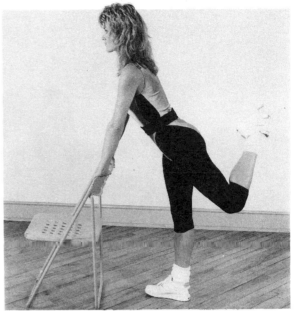

EXERCISE 3

Standing Leg Curls

8 L

PURPOSE: TO
STRENGTHEN THE
MUSCLES AT THE BACK
OF THE THIGH
(HAMSTRINGS)

16

• Face a wall or chair for support and lean slightly forwards from the hips, with hands on the wall or chair for stability

• Extend your left leg behind you, toes on the floor

• Keeping the left thigh back, slowly bend the left knee to

squeeze the heel towards the buttocks (1 count)

• Slowly lower the leg, returning the toes to the floor in the extended starting position (1 count)

• Do this 8 times slowly

□ *You should feel the back of the thigh working; if not, check that your thigh is held far enough back*

□ *Keep the hips square, and do not allow the back to arch*

□ *Keep the shoulders and left knee still*

□ *Do not lock the supporting knee*

Repeat

EXERCISE 1

Standing Side Leg Raises
6L × 2
(for your left leg) (p. 75)

32

Repeat

EXERCISE 2

Forward Squats (p. 76)
4R
(for your right leg)
Repeat

16

EXERCISE 3

Standing Leg Curls
8R
(for your right leg)
Repeat

16

EXERCISE 2

Forward Squats (p. 76)
4R + 4L
(four more times for each leg)

32

2 LEVEL

T BLOCK

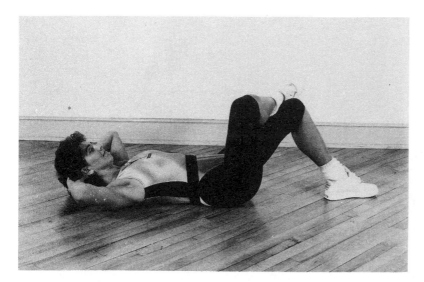

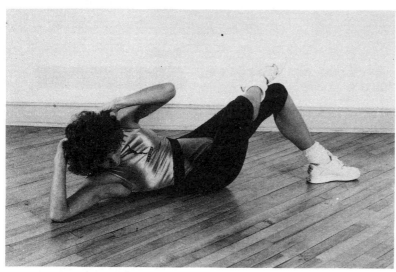

EXERCISE 4

Stomach Twists

10R

PURPOSE: TO
STRENGTHEN THE
STOMACH MUSCLES
(ABDOMINALS)

40

- Lay on your back, bend the left knee and place your left foot flat on floor

- Place both hands behind the ears to help support the head, keeping elbows out

- Place the right ankle over left knee and push the right knee out

- Keeping the stomach flat, curl your head and shoulders off the floor, twisting to the right to lean on your right elbow, taking the left elbow across to touch the right knee (2 counts). Relax (2 counts)

- Do this 10 times to the right

□ *Feel the stomach muscles working*

□ *Do not pull on your head with hands*

□ *Twist up as far as possible, keeping the lower back on the floor*

- Exercises 4-7 need to be performed on the floor. Check that you have a suitably soft covering beneath you before you start

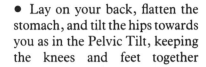

LEVEL **2**

EXERCISE 5

Buttock and Leg Squeezes

1 2

PURPOSE: TO
STRENGTHEN THE
MUSCLES OF THE INNER
THIGH (ADDUCTORS)
AND THE BUTTOCKS
(GLUTEALS)

24

- Lay on your back, flatten the stomach, and tilt the hips towards you as in the Pelvic Tilt, keeping the knees and feet together

- Lift the hips off the floor

- Squeeze the buttocks and thighs together simultaneously, then relax (2 counts)

- Do this 12 times

□ *Feel the buttocks and the inner thigh muscles working*

□ *Keep the hips still*

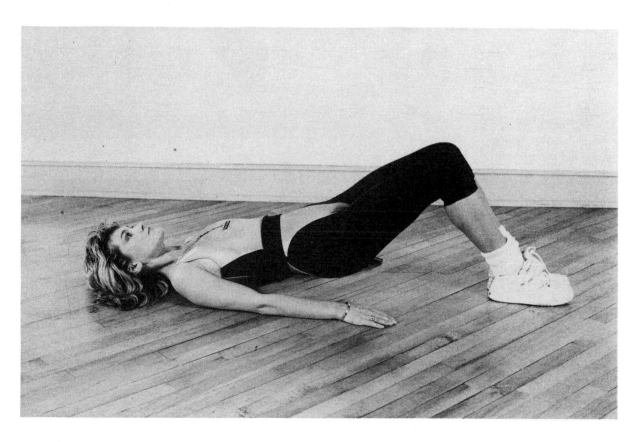

2 LEVEL

EXERCISE 6

Progressive Press-Ups

2 × 8

PURPOSE: TO STRENGTHEN THE MUSCLES AT THE BACK OF THE UPPER ARM (TRICEPS) AND THE CHEST (PECTORALS)

32

• Assume Box Press-Up position as for Level 1 (see p. 48). Move your hands about 6 inches forwards and place your shoulders directly above your hands, so that your hips move forwards beyond the knees instead of over them.

• Bend both arms, lowering your forehead to the floor and keeping the back straight, then push up (2 counts)

• Do this 8 times, rest, then repeat

□ *Feel the arms and chest working*

□ *Keep the hips high*

□ *Keep the stomach tight and the back straight*

□ *Fingers should point forwards*

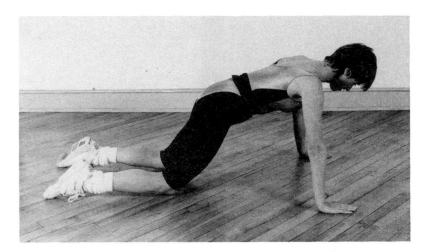

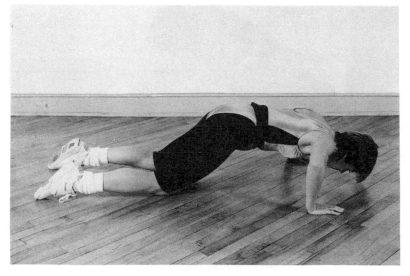

Repeat

EXERCISE 4

Stomach Twists (p. 78)
10L
(ten times to the left)
Repeat

40

EXERCISE 5

Buttock and Leg Squeezes (p. 79)
12
Repeat

24

EXERCISE 6

32

Progressive Press-Ups
2 × 28

T BLOCK

LEVEL 2

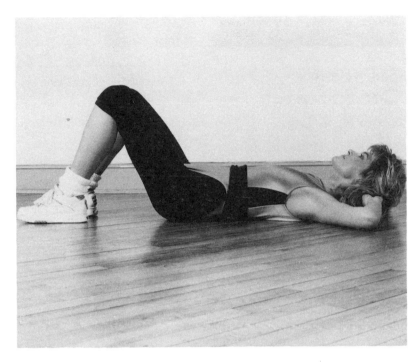

EXERCISE 7

Curl-Ups

5

PURPOSE: TO
STRENGTHEN THE
STOMACH MUSCLES
(ABDOMINALS))

10

- Lay on your back, bend both knees, with both feet flat on the floor

- Rest your head lightly in your fingertips, keeping the elbows back

- Flatten the stomach by pulling the muscles in hard, then curl head and shoulders off the floor (1 count). Relax (1 count)

- Do this 5 times

□ *Curl up to bring your shoulder blades completely off the floor and feel your stomach muscles working*

□ *Look at the tops of your knees*

□ *Do not pull on your head with your hands*

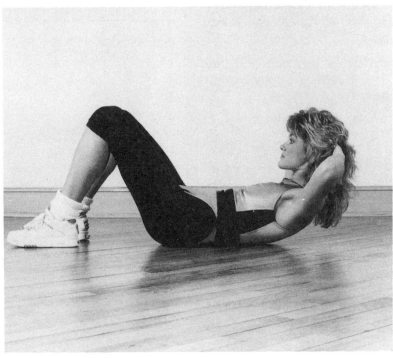

Now go on to Level 2 cool-down (p. 92)

W A R M - U P

Stretching (for aerobics)

I

minute

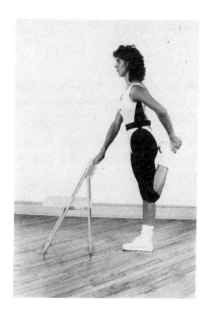

EXERCISE 1

Standing Quad Stretch

L + R

PURPOSE: TO STRETCH THE MUSCLES ALONG THE FRONT OF THE THIGH (QUADRICEPS)

16

- Face a wall or chair for support

- Transfer your weight to the right leg, bend the right knee slightly and tuck the buttocks under as for pelvic tilt

- Bring the left heel back and lift it up towards the buttocks, reaching for the left ankle with the left hand

- Use the left arm to bring the heel further up to increase the stretch

- Hold for 8 counts then repeat for the right leg

☐ *Feel the stretch down the front of the thigh*

☐ *Keep the back straight and the thighs parallel*

☐ *Maintain correct pelvic tilt*

☐ *If you don't feel a stretch, try to take the bent knee even further back*

☐ *If the bent knee is uncomfortable, try to extend the leg and the ankle will move slightly away from the body*

☐ *If you can't reach the raised ankle, loop a towel round it and gradually pull the towel upwards*

EXERCISE 2

Standing Shoulder Stretch

2

PURPOSE: TO STRETCH THE MUSCLES AROUND THE SHOULDERS

- Stand with good posture and knees slightly bent, clasp the hands together, pull in the stomach and extend the arms up above the head

- Try to pull the hands backwards to increase the stretch

- Hold for 4 counts, rest .and repeat

☐ *Feel the stretch around the shoulders*

☐ *Maintain correct pelvic tilt*

☐ *Don't arch the back*

EXERCISE 3

Standing Calf Stretch

L + R

PURPOSE: TO STRETCH THE MUSCLE ALONG THE BACK OF THE LOWER LEG (GASTROCNEMIUS)

8

- Stand with feet shoulder-width apart about three feet from a wall or chair for support, then step forward on to the right foot, bending the knee to take most of your weight, leaning on your support for balance

- Keep the left leg straight and push the heel flat to the floor

- Hold for 4 counts then repeat for the right leg

□ *Feel the stretch down the back of the lower leg*

□ *Check that both feet are facing forwards.*

□ *Check that your feet stay shoulder-width apart to aid balance*

□ *Squeeze the buttocks to stabilise the hips*

□ *If the stretch is too strong, take the front leg back and put less weight on it*

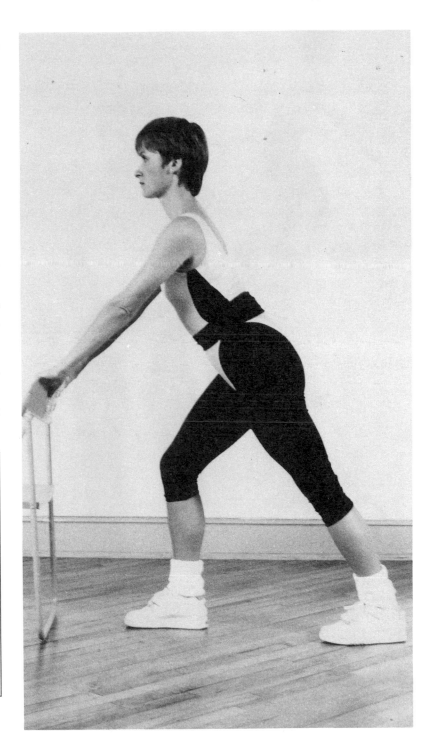

2 LEVEL

BLOCK A

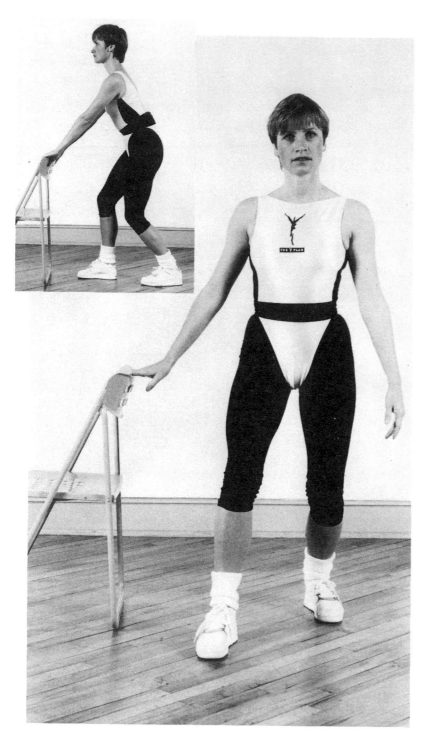

EXERCISE 4

Standing Lower Calf Stretch

L + R

PURPOSE: TO STRETCH THE MUSCLE ALONG THE BACK OF THE LOWER LEG (SOLEUS) AND THE BACK OF THE ANKLE (ACHILLES TENDON)

16

• Assume the same position as for the Standing Calf Stretch (see p. 83)

• Bring the back leg forwards a little

• Squeezing the buttocks, tilt the pelvis correctly to stabilise the hips, then bend the back leg and press the heel into the floor

• Hold for 8 counts then repeat for the right leg

□ *Feel the stretch lower down the calf of the back leg*

□ *Check that the back foot faces forwards and knee is in line with toe*

□ *Squeeze the buttocks to stabilise the hips*

□ *If you have difficulty with balance, check that your feet are not behind one another, but shoulder-width apart*

□ *Remember to take most of your weight on the back leg*

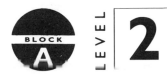

EXERCISE 5

Standing Lunge

L + R

PURPOSE: TO STRETCH
THE MUSCLES OF THE
INNER THIGH
(ADDUCTORS)

16

- Stand with feet wide apart, toes pointing slightly out

- Bend the right knee out over the right toes and slide the straight left leg away sideways, lowering the hips slightly, until you feel a stretch in the groin

- Hold for 8 counts then repeat for the right

□ *Keep both feet flat on the floor and your pelvis tucked under*

□ *Keep the hips facing front*

□ *Check your feet are wide apart*

Now begin the aerobic exercises overleaf.

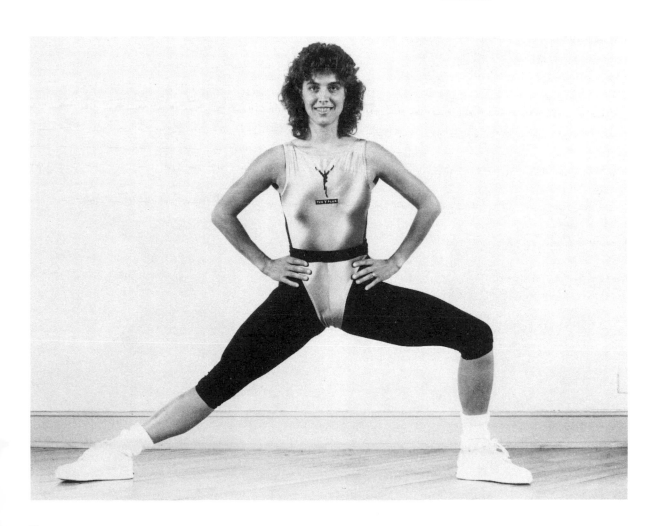

EXERCISES

(For aerobics)

The following exercises join together to form a sequence. They are designed to challenge your aerobic fitness by making your lungs and heart and circu-latory system work harder to deliver large amounts of oxygen to the working muscles. At this level you are expected to put a concerted effort into each exercise in order to work as effectively as possible. You should find your breathing rate increase during the routine and you'll feel quite warm by the end.

Should you find any exercise uncomfortable, either try to adapt it to suit you (see p. 55), miss it out altogether or find an exercise from Level 1 to complete your sequence.

If you find yourself getting quite breathless, then either take one set of exercises easily, miss out the arm movements or simply walk on the spot till you get your breath back. Try to complete the full 6 minutes on a later occasion.

6
minutes

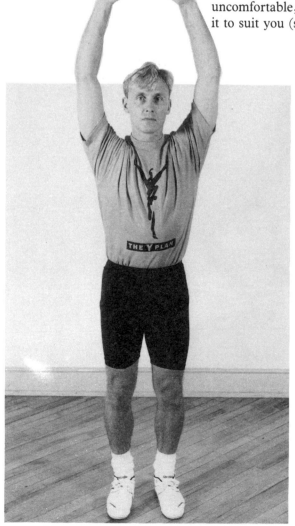

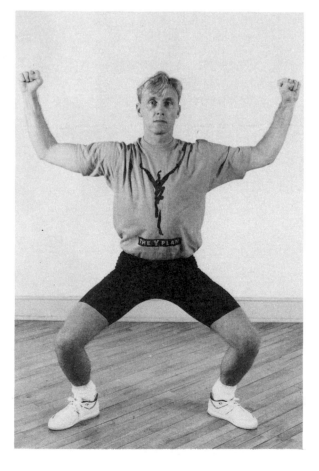

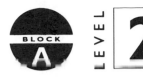

EXERCISE 1

Squat Side-Steps Adding Arm Pulls

32

4 + 4

• Stand tall with feet together and arms raised above the head

• Take a wide side-step with the right foot, bend both knees out over the toes in the squat position, simultaneously bending the elbow and pulling the arms down to shoulder height. Bring the left foot into the right, standing tall and extending the arms above the head again (2 counts)

• Repeat, taking 2 steps to the left (2 counts)

• Do this whole exercise 4 times (16 counts)

• Repeat the whole exercise 4 times again (16 counts) but with different arm movements

• Start with arms extended out in front and on the squat pull the elbows back at shoulder height and when straightening up push the arms out in front again.

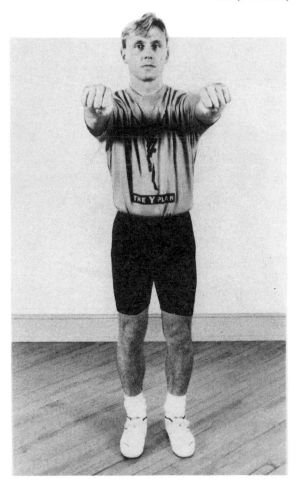

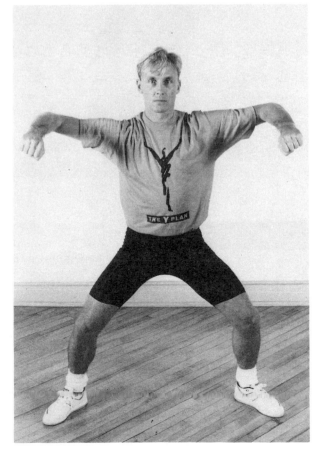

2 LEVEL BLOCK **A**

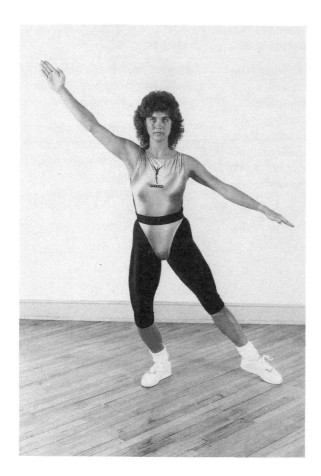

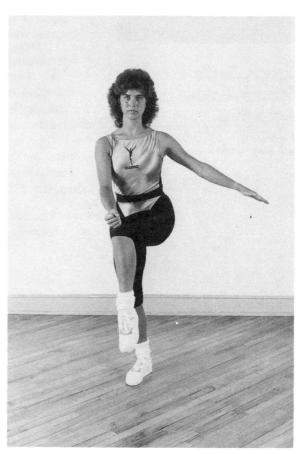

EXERCISE 2

Knee Lifts with Arm Extensions

(4R + 4L) × 2

16

- Stand with your weight on the left leg, with the right leg extended out to the side, the knee facing forward, and with your left arm extended high above your head on the left side

- Draw the right knee into the chest, bringing the left hand in to touch it, then extend the leg and arm out again (1 count)

- Do this 4 times with the right leg and 4 times with the left, then repeat

□ *Keep the stomach tight and the back straight upright*

BLOCK
A

LEVEL

2

EXERCISE 3

Digs and Skips Back

8   32

● Step forward diagonally on to the right foot, letting it take your body weight and bringing the left leg in to join the right foot, jump both feet together, bending your knees, then repeat to the left (2 counts)

● As your weight is going forwards to each side, swing your arms forwards and then back – resembling a digging action

● Skip back R, L, R, L (2 counts)

● Do the whole exercise 8 times

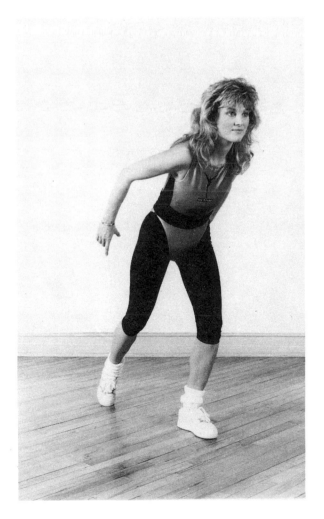

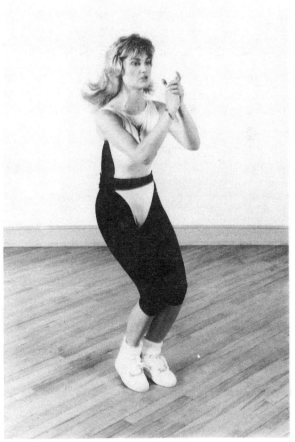

2

LEVEL

BLOCK A

EXERCISE 4

Squat Swings

16

16

- Stand on the right leg, left leg extended to the side with the toe resting on the floor

- Extend the right arm to the side just above shoulder height, with the left arm bent across the stomach

- Swing both arms to the left side of the body, simultaneously bend your legs and pass down through the squat position. Then straighten your legs and transfer your weight on to the left leg, extending the right leg to the side with the toe resting on the floor (1 count)

- Do this 16 times, alternating right and left

> ☐ *Press the heels into the floor on the squat*
>
> ☐ *Keep the bottom tucked under and the shoulders back*
>
> ☐ *Keep the back straight*

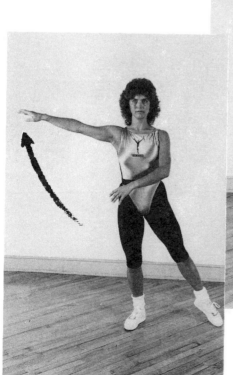
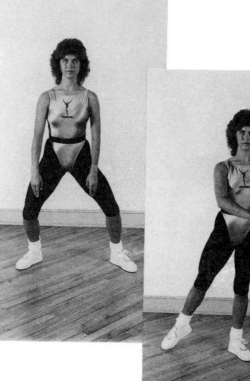

EXERCISE 5

Twists   8

8

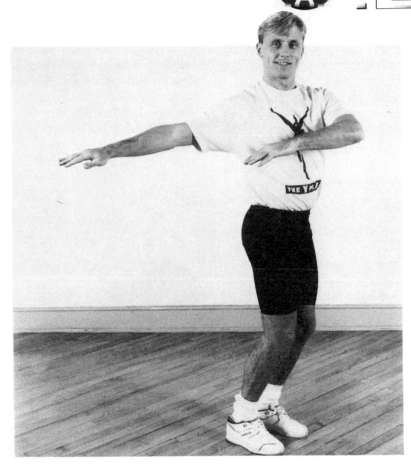

- Stand with feet hip-width apart

- Extend the right arm at shoulder height, placing the left arm bent across the chest at shoulder height

- Jump and twist shoulders to face diagonally left, feet and knees to face diagonally right, then press heels into the ground, bending the knees on landing (1 count)

- Do this 8 times, alternating right and left

EXERCISE 6

Walks with Bend and Reach   16

4

- Walk forwards 4 steps and on the fourth step bend both knees and touch the floor with both hands (2 counts)

- Walk backwards 4 steps, simultaneously reaching the arms

slowly up to the ceiling and on the fourth step, clap (2 counts)

- Do the complete exercise 4 times

□ *Don't let the buttocks go lower than the knees*

□ *Keep the head and shoulders up*

□ *If the exercise is too difficult, don't bend the knees so far*

Repeat this sequence of 6 exercises three times. Take it gently at first to give your body time to adjust. Work hard the second time, then take it easy again the third time to allow your body the chance to cool down gradually.

This whole sequence of exercises should take you 6 minutes. If you get through them in less, next time do your second sequence once or twice more.

Now go on to Level 2 cool-down overleaf.

COOL-DOWN

Again, for these exercises you need something comfortable and cushioning to work on. Breathe out as you go into the stretch and concentrate on trying to relax the muscles being stretched. In the longer stretches you can try to develop your flexibility by very gently easing even further into the stretch, but only if the tense feeling has worn off. Never bounce or jerk in your stretches; it should not be painful.

3
minutes

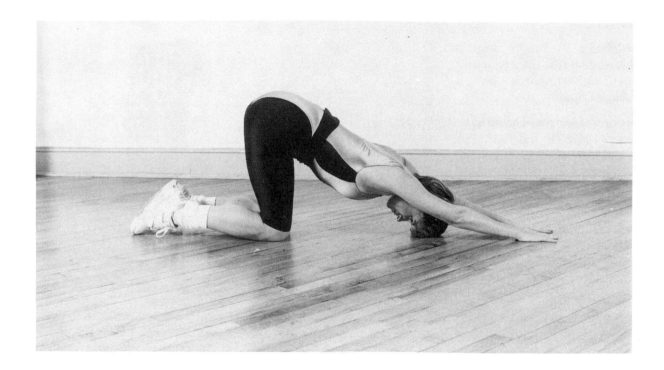

EXERCISE   1

Kneeling Shoulder Stretch

PURPOSE: TO STRETCH
THE MUSCLES AROUND
THE SHOULDERS

8

● Kneeling, sit back on your heels then lean forwards so that the chest rests on the thighs

● Extend the arms forwards and place your hands on the floor in front of you with thumbs close together

● Keeping the chest low, slide your hands and hips forwards, raising your buttocks up off your heels until your hips are directly above your knees

● Push your chest towards the floor and hold for 8 counts

☐ *Feel the stretch around your shoulders*

☐ *Keep your stomach tight to prevent the back from arching*

☐ *Look down at the floor*

T
A
BLOCK

LEVEL **2**

EXERCISE 2

Front-Lying Quad Stretch

R + L

PURPOSE: TO STRETCH THE MUSCLES ALONG THE FRONT OF THE THIGH (QUADRICEPS)

32

• On your stomach, bring the right heel in towards the buttocks

• Gently reach for the right ankle with the right hand and pull the heel in further until a stretch is felt along front of thigh

• Hold for 16 counts, developing the stretch if it eases off by lifting the knee further off the floor

• Repeat on the left

□ *Keep chin, shoulders and hips on the floor*

□ *Loop a towel round the foot if you find the ankle a little difficult to reach*

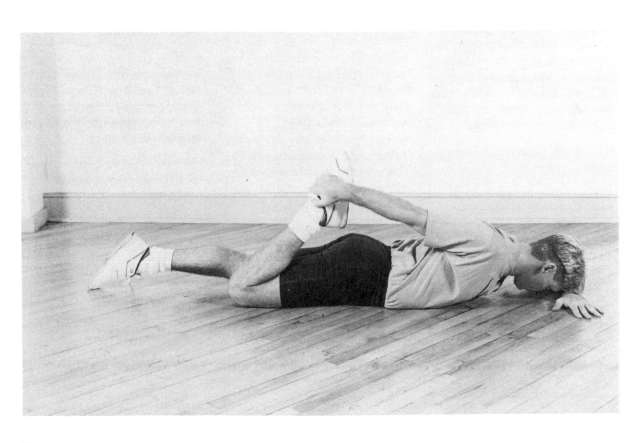

2 LEVEL **T A** BLOCK

EXERCISE 3

Lying Stomach Stretch

2

PURPOSE: TO STRETCH THE STOMACH MUSCLES (ABDOMINALS) AND TO MOBILISE THE SPINE

16

● Lie on your front and place your hands flat on the floor in front of your head, with arms slightly bent(see p. 59)

● Gently lift the head and shoulders off the floor by pushing on your hands and extending your arms. Keeping your hips on the floor, walk your hands back towards you until you feel a stretch down your stomach

● Hold for 8 counts, relax then repeat

☐ *Pull your stomach in to increase the stretch*

☐ *Look ahead and keep your hip bones on the floor*

☐ *If your back aches, lower your shoulders further or leave this exercise out*

☐ *Think of lengthening your spine*

EXERCISE 4

Sitting Hamstring Stretch

L + R

PURPOSE: TO STRETCH THE MUSCLES AT THE BACK OF THE THIGH (HAMSTRINGS)

48

● Sit on the floor, with left leg straight out in front and right leg slightly to the side, bent out of the way (see p. 71)

● Sit up tall and place your hands on the floor either side of your left leg

● Pull in the stomach and, trying to keep your back straight, bend forwards over the straight leg until you feel the stretch down the back of the left leg

● Hold for 24 counts, increasing the stretch if it eases off by lowering the chest nearer to the straight leg

● Repeat for the right leg

☐ *Keep the hips square*

☐ *Ease down gently*

☐ *Don't be competitive. It is not necessary to rest your head on your leg*

☐ *This should not be felt in your back. If it is, try the Lying Hamstring stretch, on p. 62*

EXERCISE 5

Sitting Groin Stretch

PURPOSE: TO STRETCH THE MUSCLES OF THE INNER THIGH (ADDUCTORS)

16

● Sit on the floor and bring the soles of the feet together as close to the groin as possible (see (p. 61)

● Place a hand on each ankle and press the knees towards the floor with the elbows until you feel a stretch in the groin

● Hold for 16 counts, trying to relax the muscles. If you feel the stretch becomes easier, press down with the elbows a little more to develop the stretch and improve flexibility

☐ *Sit up as straight as possible*

☐ *Keep the shoulders down*

EXERCISE 6

Standing Side Stretch

L + R

PURPOSE: TO STRETCH
THE MUSCLES IN THE
SIDE OF THE BODY

16

- Stand with feet shoulder-width apart, knees slightly bent and with correct pelvic tilt

- Place the right hand on the right hip, with the left arm extended above your head

- Pull the stomach in tight and bend slowly to the right, keeping the body facing forwards, extending the left arm up and over to the right diagonal until you feel a stretch down the left side

- Hold for 8 counts then repeat on the other side

□ *Breathe out on the stretch*

□ *Keep your shoulders in line with your hips*

□ *Keep your arm and head in line with the shoulders*

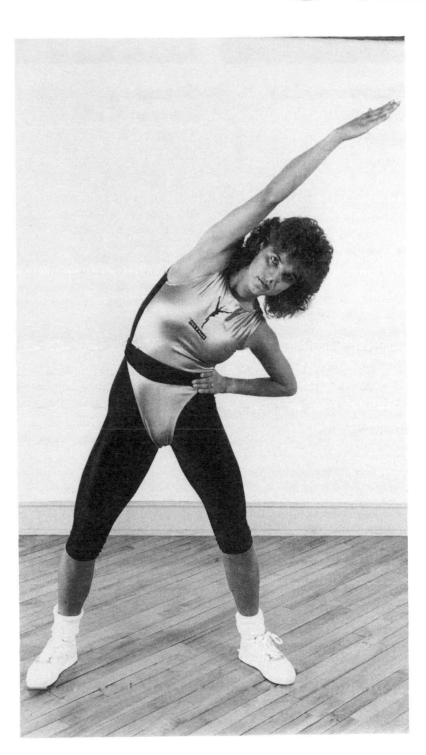

2 LEVEL T/A BLOCK

EXERCISE 7

Standing Calf Stretch

L + R

PURPOSE: TO STRETCH THE MUSCLE ALONG THE BACK OF THE LOWER LEG (GASTROCNEMIUS) 16

● Stand with feet shoulder-width apart about three feet from a wall or chair for support, then step forward on to the right foot, bending the knee to take most of your weight, leaning on your support for balance (see p. 83)

● Keep the left leg straight and push the heel flat to the floor

● Hold for 8 counts then repeat for the right leg

> ☐ Feel a stretch down the back of the lower leg
>
> ☐ Check that both feet are facing forwards.
>
> ☐ If the stretch is too strong, take the front leg back and put less weight on it
>
> ☐ Check that your feet stay shoulder-width apart to aid balance
>
> ☐ Squeeze the buttocks to stabilise the hips

EXERCISE 8

Standing Lower Calf Stretch

L + R

PURPOSE: TO STRETCH THE MUSCLE ALONG THE BACK OF THE LOWER LEG (SOLEUS) AND THE BACK OF THE ANKLE (ACHILLES TENDON) 16

● Assume the same position as for the Standing Calf Stretch (see p. 83)

● Bring the back leg forwards a little

● Squeezing the buttocks, tilt the pelvis correctly to stabilise the hips, then bend the back leg and press the heel into the floor

● Hold for 8 counts then repeat for the right leg

> ☐ Feel the stretch lower down the calf of the back leg
>
> ☐ Check that the back foot faces forwards and knee is in line with toe
>
> ☐ Squeeze the buttocks to stabilise the hips
>
> ☐ If you have difficulty with balance, check that your feet are not behind one another, but shoulder-width apart
>
> ☐ Remember to take most of your weight on the back leg

EXERCISE 9

Standing Chest Stretch

2

PURPOSE: TO STRETCH THE MUSCLES ACROSS THE FRONT OF THE CHEST (PECTORALS) 12

● Stand with good posture and knees slightly bent, clasping hands together behind the back (see p. 74)

● Extend the arms out and up behind the back

● Hold for 6 counts, rest and repeat

> ☐ Feel the stretch across the front of the chest
>
> ☐ Maintain correct pelvic tilt and don't bend forwards

WARM-UP

The warm-up section is divided into two parts.

The first two minutes are always done regardless of whether your main exercise block

on a given day is for toning or aerobics.

You then follow this with one minute of stretching for either the toning warm-up or the aerobic warm-up. After completing the appropriate warm-up, you go on to six minutes of toning or aerobic exercise, followed by the three-minute cool-down.

Mobility and pulse-raising (for muscle toning and aerobics)

Remember that you can speed up the exercises by counting 'one and' a bit faster.

2
minutes

EXERCISE 1

Step Tap with Arms

16

PURPOSE: TO LOOSEN THE JOINTS, TO GENERATE HEAT AND WARM THE MUSCLES

16

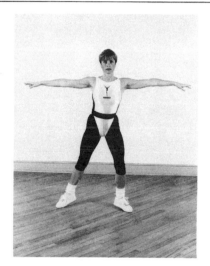
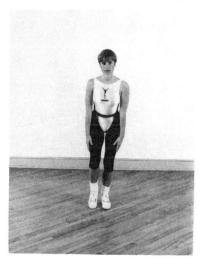
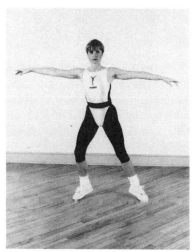
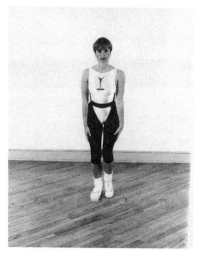

- Step sideways on to the right foot and tap the left foot next to it with a little knee-bend, lifting the arms straight out to the sides at shoulder height on the step and bringing them down to slap the thighs on the tap

- Repeat on the left leg (1 count)

- Do this complete exercise 8 times, alternating right and left

3 LEVEL

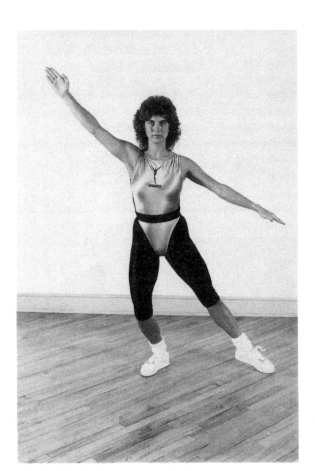

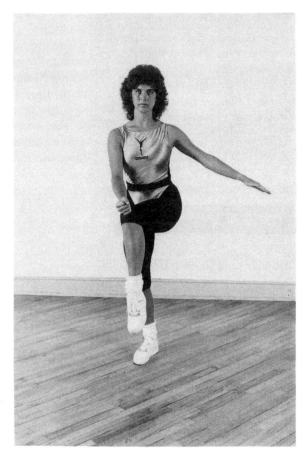

EXERCISE 2

Knee Lifts with Arm Extensions

(4R + 4L) × 2

PURPOSE: TO GENERATE HEAT AND WARM THE MUSCLES

16

- Stand with your weight on the left leg, with the right leg extended out to the side with the knee facing forward, and with the left arm extended high above your head on the left side

- Draw the right knee into the chest, bringing the left hand in to touch it, then extend the leg and arm out again (1 count)

- Do this 4 times with the right leg and 4 times with the left, then repeat

> □ *Keep the stomach tight and the back straight upright*

BLOCK T A

LEVEL **3**

EXERCISE 3

Leg Tap Out with Arm Swings

(4R + 4L) × 2

PURPOSE: TO GENERATE
HEAT AND WARM THE
MUSCLES

16

- Bend left leg, with arms bent and crossed in front of your body. Keep your weight on the left leg

- Straighten the right leg out to the right, knee facing forward, and tap your toe on the floor. Bring it back to tap the floor next to your left foot. Simultaneously swing both arms out to shoulder height as you extend the right leg, and back in front of your body as you close (1 count)

- Do this 4 times with the right leg and 4 times with the left, then repeat

☐ *Keep the stomach tight and lean very slightly forwards from the hips*

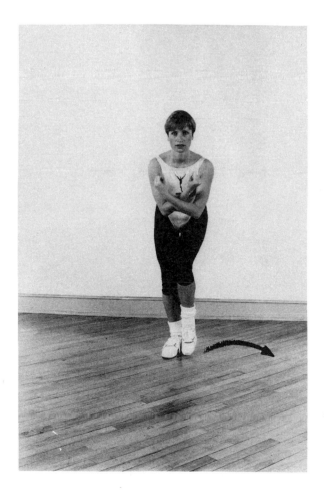

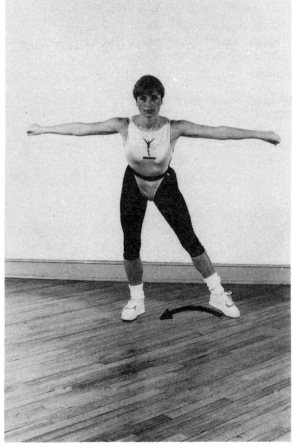

3 LEVEL

T
BLOCK
A

EXERCISE 4

Waist Twists

8

PURPOSE: TO MOBILISE
THE WAIST AND BACK

16

• Stand with good posture, knees slightly bent

• Squeeze the buttocks and tighten the stomach

• Keeping the hips still, gently twist your shoulders and head round to the right, return to centre (2 counts). Repeat to the left and return to centre (2 counts)

• Do this complete exercise 4 times

☐ *Keep the hips facing front*

☐ *Move round slowly, keeping the back upright*

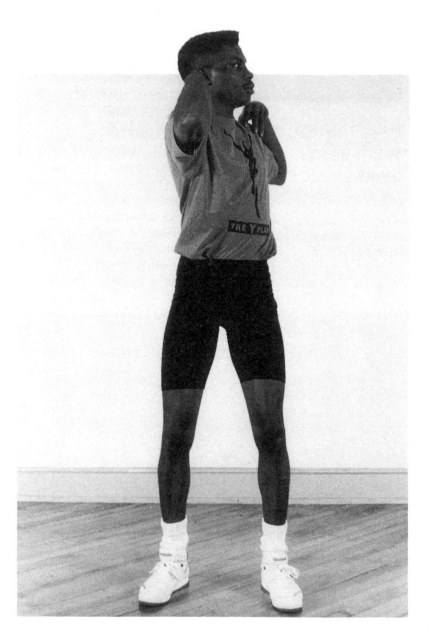

EXERCISE 5

Double Arm Circles

8

PURPOSE: TO GENERATE
HEAT, WARM THE
MUSCLES AND MOBILISE
THE SHOULDERS

16

• Stand with good posture

• Extend both arms out to the front and circle them forwards, up and over behind your head (2 counts)

• Do this 8 times

☐ *Take the arms back close to your ears*

☐ *Take the movement slowly*

EXERCISE · 6

Ankle Circles
4R + 4L

PURPOSE: TO MOBILISE
THE ANKLES

8

● Stand on the left leg, place the right toes on the floor near the left foot (see p. 34)

● Circle the right ankle 4 times, taking it forwards then out, back and round (4 counts)

● Repeat this 4 times with the left ankle (4 counts)

□ *Feel the movement in the ankles*

□ *Keep the hips still*

Repeat

EXERCISE · 2

Knee Lifts with Arm Extensions (p. 98)
(4R + 4L) × 2

16
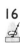

Repeat

EXERCISE · 3

Leg Tap Out with Arm Swings (p. 99)
(4R + 4L) × 2

16

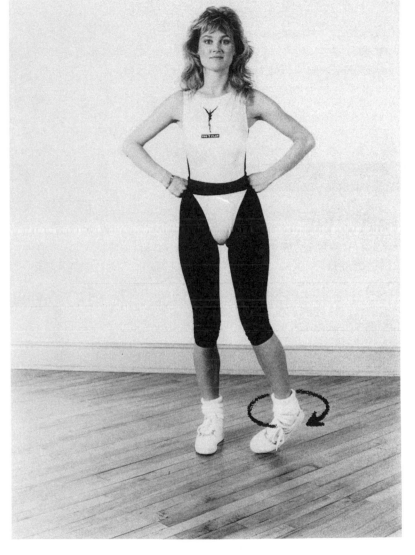

Now go on to either the one-minute toning warm-up stretch overleaf or the one - minute aerobic warm-up stretch on p. 112, depending on which seven-and-a-half-minute block you are doing.

3 LEVEL

WARM - UP

Stretching (for muscle toning)

Some stretches are only held for a short time. Be sure to perform them effectively.

|
minute

EXERCISE | 1

Rear Bent Arm Shoulder Stretch

R + L

PURPOSE: TO STRETCH THE MUSCLE AROUND THE SHOULDER (DELTOID)

16

• Stand with good posture, bend the right arm and take the right hand up behind your back, between the shoulder blades

• Try to grasp the right elbow behind with the left hand and ease the right elbow across to the left to increase stretch

• Hold for 8 counts and repeat with the left elbow

☐ *Feel the stretch down the side of your shoulder*

☐ *Grasp the wrist if you cannot reach the elbow and ease it across to the side*

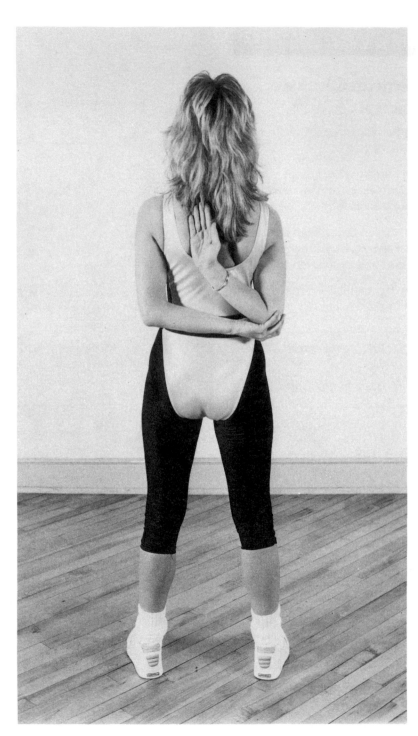

EXERCISE 2

Standing Triceps Stretch

L + R

PURPOSE: TO STRETCH THE MUSCLE ALONG THE BACK OF THE UPPER ARM (TRICEPS)

16

• Stand with good posture and knees slightly bent, curve the left arm behind the head and place the fingers on the upper back between the shoulder blades (see p. 70)

• Using the right hand, assist the stretch by gently pulling the left elbow across behind your head

• Hold for 8 counts then repeat for the right arm

□ *Feel the stretch down the back of the upper arm*

EXERCISE 3

Standing Hamstring Stretch

R + L

PURPOSE: TO STRETCH THE MUSCLES AT THE BACK OF THE THIGH (HAMSTRINGS)

16

• Gently raise the hips, by extending the right leg and transferring your weight back on to the left leg until you feel a stretch down the back of the right leg

• Hold for 8 counts and repeat on the left

□ *Keep your chest on your thigh to protect your back. Your legs will not be and do not need to be straight*

□ *Check that the back knee does not roll inwards; keep it over the toe*

• Stand with your feet just over shoulder-width apart and knees bent

• Turn your body and toes diagonally to the right

• Pull the stomach in to support your back and bend forwards to rest your chest on the right thigh, keeping your weight evenly balanced between your feet

• Hold the right lower leg with both hands for support

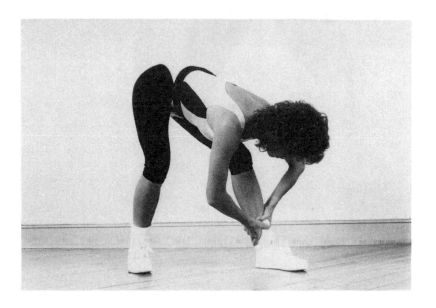

3 LEVEL

T
BLOCK

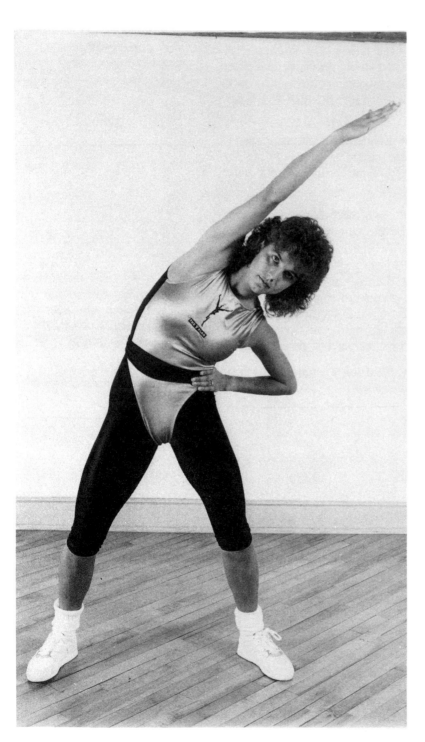

EXERCISE 4

Standing Side Stretch

L + R

PURPOSE: TO STRETCH
THE MUSCLES IN THE
SIDE OF THE BODY

8

• Stand with feet shoulder-width apart, knees slightly bent and with correct pelvic tilt

• Place the right hand on the right hip, with the left arm extended above your head

• Pull the stomach in tight and bend slowly to the right, keeping the body facing forwards, extending the left arm up and over to the right diagonal until you feel a stretch down the left side

• Hold for 4 counts then repeat on the other side

□ *Breathe out on the stretch*

□ *Keep your shoulders in line with your hips*

□ *Keep your arm and head in line with the shoulders*

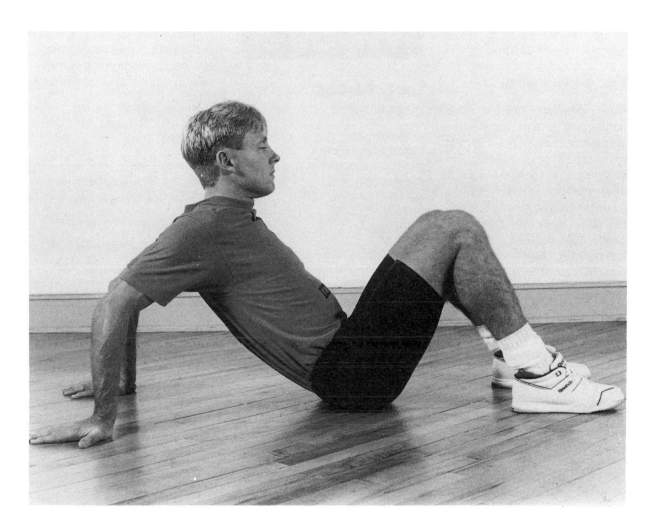

EXERCISE 5

Sitting Shoulder Stretch

PURPOSE: TO STRETCH
THE MUSCLES AROUND
THE FRONT PART OF THE
SHOULDERS (DELTOIDS)

8

- Sit on the floor with legs bent, both feet flat and both hands flat on the floor behind you, fingers pointing away from your body

- Bend the elbows slightly and slide your bottom away from your hands until you feel a stretch in the front of the shoulders

- Hold for 8 counts

□ *Keep the elbows bent*

□ *Place your hands near together*

Now begin the muscle toning exercises overleaf.

E X E R C I S E S

(For muscle toning)

These exercises will be quite demanding at first. Ensure that your exercise technique is correct and stop if your muscles feel fatigued, as you will no longer be able to perform correctly. Breathe out on the effort and work through the full range of movement. Check that you have something comfortable and cushioning beneath you to work on.

7½
minutes

EXERCISE 1

Leg Raises
16R + 16L

PURPOSE: TO STRENGTHEN THE MUSCLES AT THE BACK OF THE THIGH (HAMSTRINGS) AND OF THE BUTTOCKS (GLUTEALS)

64

• Position yourself on hands and knees (box position) with your hands under your shoulders and the hips over the knees, then extend the right leg out behind, toes on the floor

• Keeping the stomach tight and the lower back still, raise the right leg straight till level with the hips, then lower back down to the floor (2 counts)

• Do this 16 times, then repeat on the left

□ *Feel the muscles at the back of the thigh working*

□ *Look between your hands*

□ *Keep the arms straight*

□ *Keep the hips square to the floor*

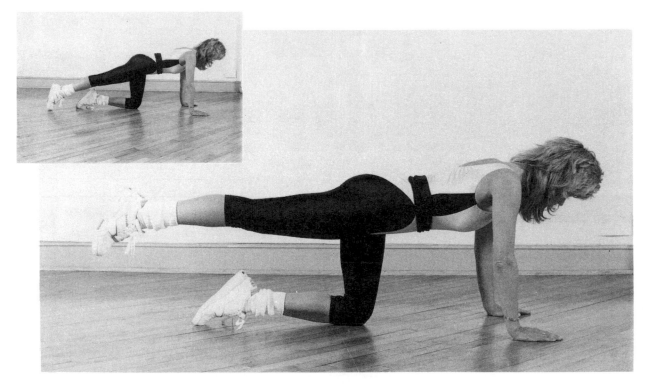

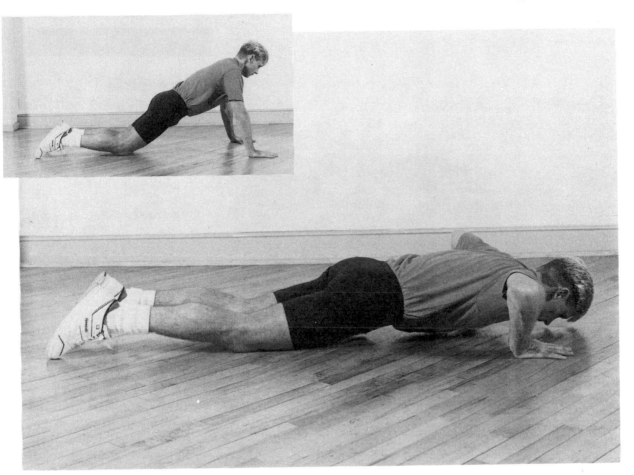

EXERCISE   2

Intermediate Press-Ups

12 + 16

PURPOSE: TO
STRENGTHEN THE
MUSCLES AT THE BACK
OF THE UPPER ARM
(TRICEPS) AND ACROSS
THE CHEST (PECTORALS)

64

● With hands and knees on the floor, place your shoulder over your hands and your knees far enough back for your body to be in a straight line from knees to shoulders

● Bend both arms to lower the body, so that thighs, hips, chest and nose touch the floor simultaneously, then return to start (2 counts)

● Do this 12 times, rest for 8 counts then repeat 16 times

□ *Feel the chest and upper arm muscles working*

□ *Tilt the pelvis to prevent your back from hollowing*

□ *Keep the shoulders over the hands*

If this is uncomfortable, go back to either the Box Press-Ups (p. 48) or the Progressive Press-Ups (p. 80).

3 LEVEL **T** BLOCK

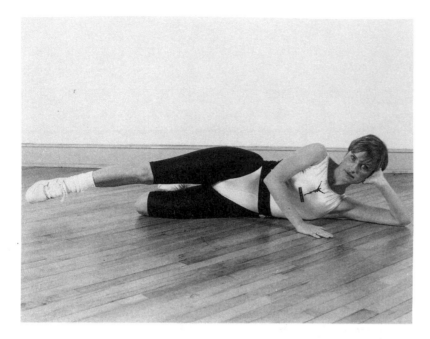

EXERCISE 3

Lying Side Leg Raises

16L

PURPOSE: TO
STRENGTHEN THE
MUSCLES AT THE SIDE
OF THE HIP
(ABDUCTORS)

32

• Lie on your right side, keeping the thighs together and the hips straight. Bend the right leg for stability

• Place your left hand on the floor in front of your chest for support and rest your head in your right hand

• Keeping the hips still and facing forwards, raise the left leg straight as far as possible, keeping the knee facing forwards, then lower (2 counts)

• Do this 16 times

☐ *Feel the outside of your leg and hip working*

☐ *Keep the body straight*

☐ *Keep the hips straight; do not lean back*

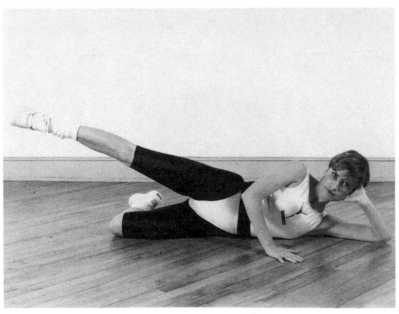

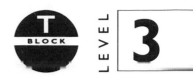

LEVEL **3**

EXERCISE 4

Twisting Curl-Ups with Leg Extensions

16L

PURPOSE: TO
STRENGTHEN THE
STOMACH MUSCLES
(ABDOMINALS) AND THE
HIP FLEXORS

32

● Lie on your back with your hands behind the ears, right leg bent with the right foot flat on the floor for support, and the left leg extended upwards parallel with the right thigh

● Press your lower back into the floor and flatten the stomach by tilting the pelvis correctly

● Curl your head and shoulders off the floor while bringing the left knee in and twisting your body to the left so that your right

elbow meets the left knee (1 count), then relax and extend the left leg again (1 count)

● Do this 16 times

□ *Feel your stomach muscles working*

□ *Keep the lower back on the floor throughout the exercise*

□ *Do not pull on your head*

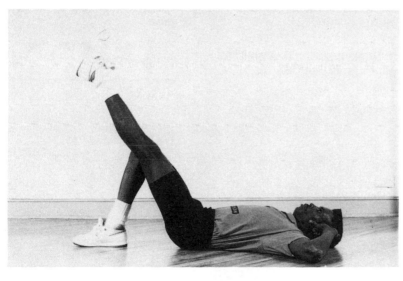

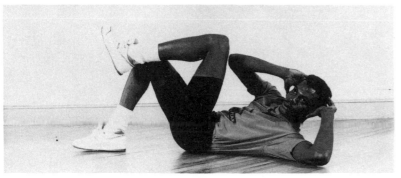

Repeat

EXERCISE 3

Lying Side Leg Raises (p. 108)
16L
(on the left leg again)

32

Repeat

EXERCISE 4

Twisting Curl-Ups with Leg Extensions
16R
(using the right leg and twisting to the right)
Repeat

32

EXERCISE 3

Lying Side Leg Raises (p. 108)
16R
(now on the right leg)

32

3 LEVEL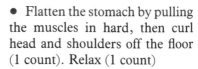

EXERCISE 5

Curl-Ups with Leg Extensions

8R + 8L

PURPOSE: TO
STRENGTHEN THE
STOMACH MUSCLES
(ABDOMINALS) AND THE
HIP FLEXORS

32

● Lie on your back, with your hands behind the ears, left leg bent with the left foot flat on the floor for support, and the right leg extended upwards parallel with the left thigh (see p. 109)

● Press your lower back into the floor and flatten the stomach by tilting the pelvis correctly

● Curl the head and shoulders off the floor while bringing the right leg in to meet both elbows (1 count), then relax and extend the leg again (1 count)

● Do this 8 times then repeat with the left leg 8 times

□ *Feel the stomach muscles working*

□ *Remember not to twist when curling up*

□ *Keep the lower back on the floor throughout the exercise*

□ *Do not pull on your head*

□ *Always keep one leg bent with the foot flat on the floor*

Repeat

EXERCISE 3

*Lying Side Leg Raises
(p. 108)*
16R
(again on the right leg)

32

EXERCISE 6

Curl-Ups

16

PURPOSE: TO
STRENGTHEN THE
STOMACH MUSCLES
(ABDOMINALS)

● Lay on your back, bend both knees, with both feet flat on the floor

● Rest your head lightly in your fingertips, keeping the elbows back

● Flatten the stomach by pulling the muscles in hard, then curl head and shoulders off the floor (1 count). Relax (1 count)

● Do this 16 times

□ *Curl up to bring your shoulder blades completely off the floor and feel your stomach muscles working*

□ *Look at the tops of your knees*

□ *Do not pull on your head with your hands*

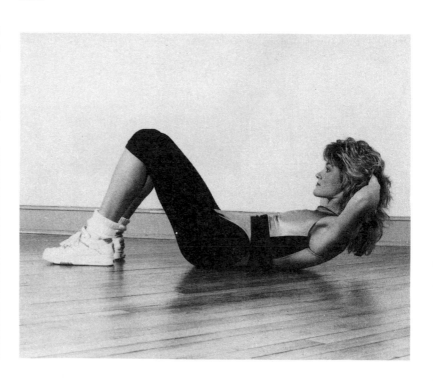

EXERCISE· 7

Dips and Squeezes

(8S + 8F) × 2

PURPOSE: TO
STRENGTHEN THE
MUSCLES AT THE BACK
OF THE UPPER ARMS
(TRICEPS), THE MUSCLES
OF THE INNER THIGHS
(ADDUCTORS) AND THE
BUTTOCKS (GLUTEALS)

32

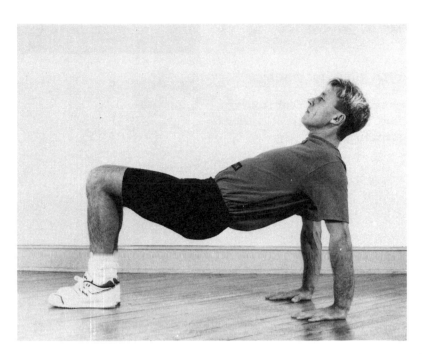

• Sit up with legs bent and held together and both feet flat on the floor. Place both hands on the floor behind you with fingers pointing forwards

• Lift your hips off the floor, making sure that both shoulders are directly over your hands, and your knees are directly over your feet

• Bend the arms, lowering the shoulders towards the floor (1 count). Extend the arms, squeezing knees and buttocks together (1 count)

• Do this 8 times slowly (bend + extend = 2 counts) then 8 times fast (bend + extend = 1 count). Rest for 8 counts then repeat 8 times slowly and 8 times fast, and rest for 8 counts

□ *Feel the arm muscles working*

□ *Try to avoid dropping the hips*

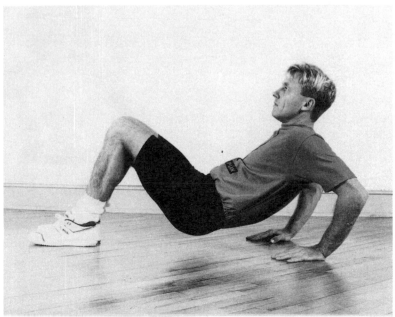

Now go on to Level 3 cool-down (p. 123).

WARM-UP

Stretching (for aerobics)

Some stretches are only held for a short time. Be sure to perform them effectively.

I

minute

EXERCISE I

Standing Lunge

L + R

PURPOSE: TO STRETCH THE MUSCLES OF THE INNER THIGH (ADDUCTORS)

16

- Stand with feet wide apart, toes pointing slightly out

- Bend the right knee out over the right toes and slide the straight left leg away sideways, lowering the hips slightly, until you feel a stretch in the groin

- Hold for 8 counts then repeat for the left

□ *Keep both feet flat on the floor and your pelvis tucked under*

□ *Keep the hips facing front*

□ *Check your feet are wide apart*

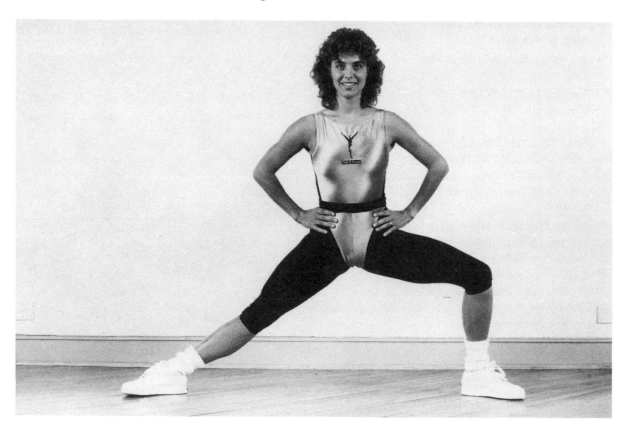

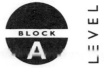

EXERCISE 2

Standing Hamstring Stretch

R + L

PURPOSE: TO STRETCH THE MUSCLES AT THE BACK OF THE THIGH (HAMSTRINGS)

16

• Stand with your feet just over shoulder-width apart and knees bent (see p. 103)

• Turn your body and toes diagonally to the right

• Pull the stomach in to support your back and bend forwards to rest your chest on the right thigh, keeping your weight evenly balanced between your feet

• Hold the right lower leg with both hands for support

• Gently raise the hips, by extending the right leg and transferring your weight back on to the left leg until you feel a stretch down the back of the right leg

• Hold for 8 counts and repeat on the left

> □ *Keep your chest on your thigh to protect your back. Your legs will not be and do not need to be straight*
>
> □ *Check that the back knee does not roll inwards; keep it over the toe*

EXERCISE 3

Standing Side Stretch

L + R

PURPOSE: TO STRETCH THE MUSCLES IN THE SIDE OF THE BODY

8

• Stand with feet shoulder-width apart, knees slightly bent and with correct pelvic tilt (see p. 104)

• Place the right hand on the right hip, with the left arm extended above your head

• Pull the stomach in tight and bend slowly to the right, keeping the body facing forwards, extending the left arm up and over to the right diagonal until you feel a stretch down the left side

• Hold for 4 counts then repeat on the other side

> □ *Breathe out on the stretch*
>
> □ *Keep your shoulders in line with your hips*
>
> □ *Keep the arm and head in line with the shoulders*

EXERCISE 4

Standing Quad Stretch

L + R

PURPOSE: TO STRETCH THE MUSCLES ALONG THE FRONT OF THE THIGH (QUADRICEPS)

8

• Stand on your right leg, bend the right knee slightly and tuck the buttocks under as for pelvic tilt (see p. 72)

• Bring the left heel back and up towards the buttocks, reaching for the left ankle with the left hand to bring the heel further up so as to increase the stretch.

• Hold for 4 counts then repeat for the right leg

> □ *Feel the stretch down the front of the thigh*
>
> □ *Stretch the free arm out to the side to assist balance*
>
> □ *Keep the back straight and the thighs parallel*
>
> □ *Maintain correct pelvic tilt*
>
> □ *If you don't feel a stretch, try to take the bent knee even further back*
>
> □ *If the bent knee is uncomfortable, try to extend the leg and the ankle will move slightly away from the body*

3 LEVEL

BLOCK
A

EXERCISE 5

Bridge Calf Stretch

R + L

PURPOSE: TO STRETCH
THE MUSCLE ALONG THE
BACK OF THE LOWER LEG
(GASTROCNEMIUS)

8

• Position yourself with hands and feet shoulder-width apart on the floor and hips pointing in the air, looking at the floor between your hands (bridge position)

• With the left leg slightly bent and the right leg straight, press the right heel into the floor so as to feel a stretch in the calf

• Hold for 4 counts then repeat on the left

☐ *Push the heel down hard, point the toes forwards and keep the stretched leg straight*

☐ *Adjust the distance between hands and feet to increase the stretch; the closer together the harder the stretch*

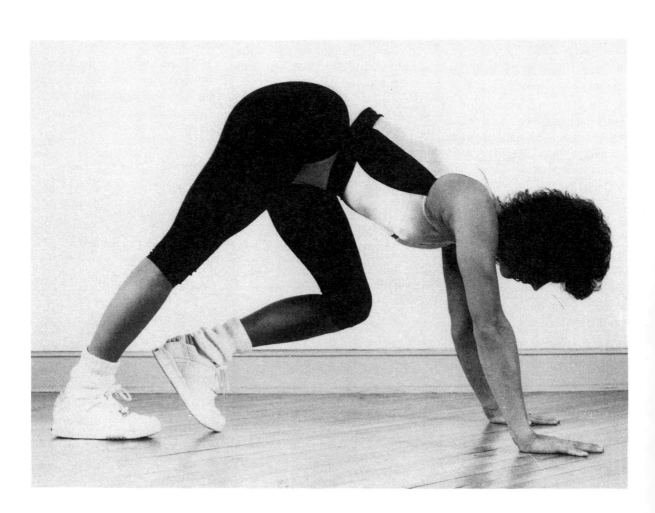

LEVEL 3

EXERCISE 6

Bridge Lower Calf Stretch
R + L

PURPOSE: TO STRETCH THE MUSCLE ALONG THE BACK OF THE LOWER LEG (SOLEUS) AND THE BACK OF THE ANKLE (ACHILLES TENDON)

8

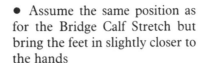

• Assume the same position as for the Bridge Calf Stretch but bring the feet in slightly closer to the hands

• Bend both legs slightly and press the heel of the right leg into the floor

• Hold for 4 counts then repeat on the left

□ *Feel the stretch lower down the calf*

□ *Transfer your weight back over the heel to increase the stretch*

Now begin the aerobic exercises overleaf.

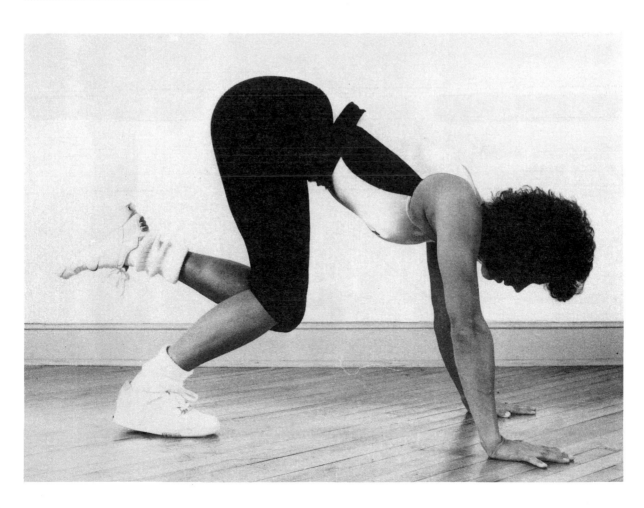

E X E R C I S E S

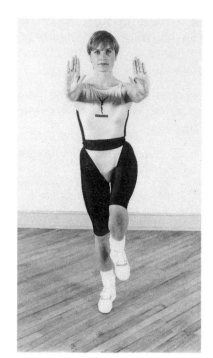

(For aerobics)

The following exercises combine to make a challenging sequence. Try to find your own rhythm that enables you to keep the exercises moving continuously. If you want to work harder, extend all the movements, making them as big as you can. This will be a demanding sequence once you have mastered the exercises.

7½
minutes

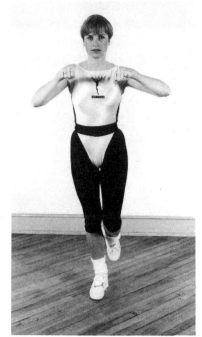

E X E R C I S E   I

Marches with Arm Pushes 16
(I + I) × 2

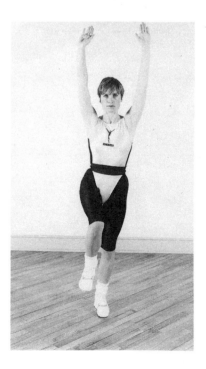

- March on the spot for 4 counts (R + L = 1 count) and swing arms vigorously

- March on the spot again, bending and extending the arms out in front from the chest once, once above the head, once out in front, and once above the head (4 counts)

- Repeat both exercises

> □ *Lift the knees high on marches*

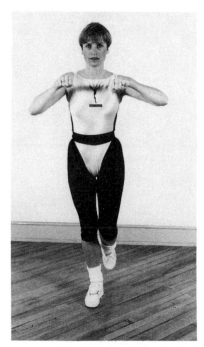

116

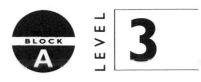

EXERCISE 2

Jog on the Spot and Clap

8   8

● Jog on the spot for 8 counts (R + L = 1 count) lifting the heels to touch the buttocks and simul-taneously extending the arms to each side, then clapping in front on every count

☐ *Keep the arms at shoulder height*

☐ *Push the heels into the floor*

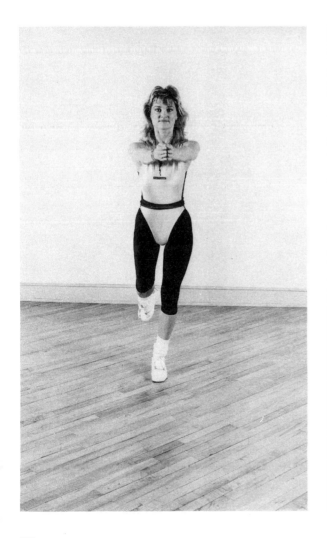

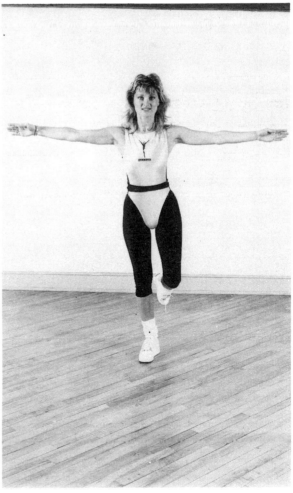

3 LEVEL BLOCK **A**

EXERCISE 3

Squat and Reach

4   8

![icon]

• Stand with feet shoulder-width apart, clap once and squat, slapping hands on bent knees (1 count; see p. 67)

• Straighten legs, clapping hands in front and then reaching your arms high to the ceiling (1 count)

• Do this complete exercise 4 times

□ *Keep the back straight and upright*

□ *Push the knees out over feet on the squat*

□ *Really stretch up on the reaches*

Repeat

EXERCISE 2

Jog on the Spot and Clap (p. 117)
8   8

![icon]

Repeat

EXERCISE 3

Squat and Reach
4   8

![icon]

EXERCISE 4

Jumping Knee Lifts with Arm Pulls and Ski Swings   16

(1 + 1) × 4   ![icon]

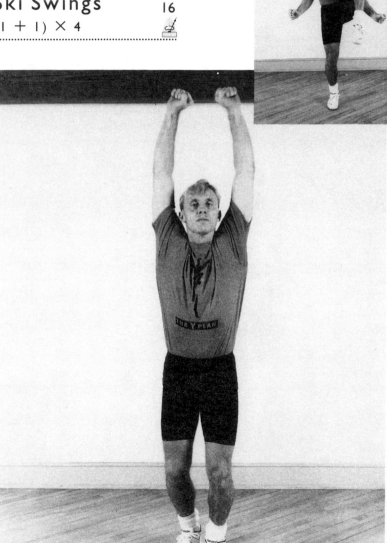

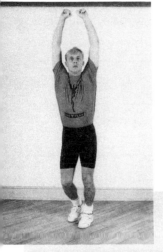

- Stand with feet hip-width apart and arms stretched above the head

- Hop on to the left leg, lifting the right knee to the chest and pulling elbows down into the waist, then jump to join the feet together, extending both arms up again above your head then repeat on the right leg (2 counts)

- With both feet on the floor and parallel, bend the knees, then straighten again simultaneously swinging the arms down past the thighs and back as far as they will go, then bend the knees and straighten again while the arms swing forwards and up (2 counts)

- Do both exercises 4 times

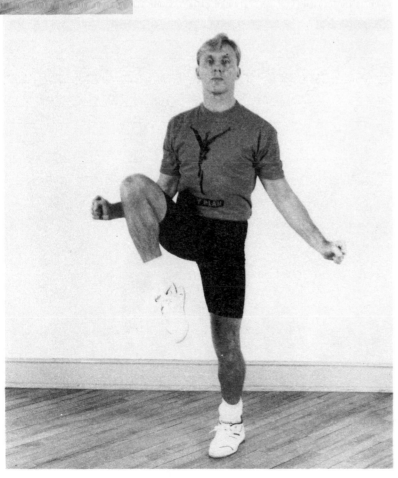

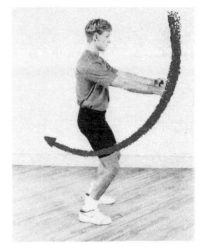

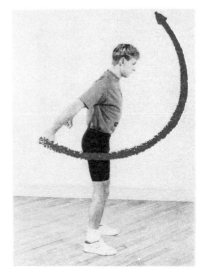

3 LEVEL BLOCK A

EXERCISE 5

Side to Side Jumps with Arm Swings

4

4

....

• Start with feet together then jump-turn to the right, landing

with feet about 18 inches apart, the right foot in front of the left, then jump-turn back to the centre, feet together and facing forwards

• At the same time, swing both arms straight up above your head when feet jump-land apart and bring both arms down to the sides when feet jump-land together (1 count)

• Do this complete exercise with a jump-turn to the left and centre (1 count)

• Repeat once more, to the right and left

☐ *Keep your knees in line with your toes*

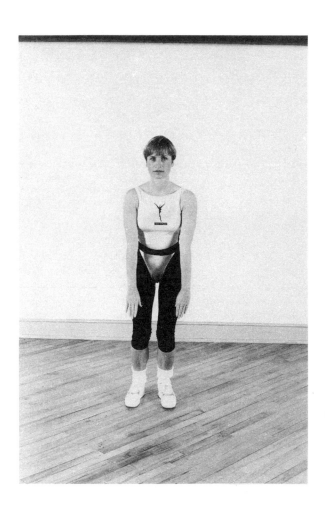

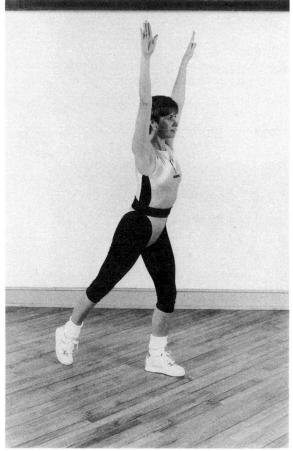

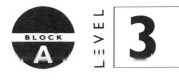

EXERCISE 6

Knee Lifts with Arm Pulls

4   4

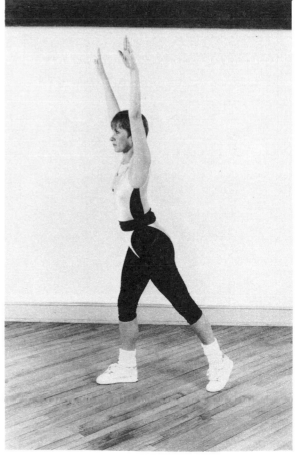

• Stand on your left leg with both arms extended above your head. Lift the right knee to the chest, pulling the elbows down into the waist then straighten (1 count; see p. 118, without the jump)

• Repeat with the left knee (1 count)

• Do this once more, on the right and left

> ☐ *Keep the back straight on the knee lifts*

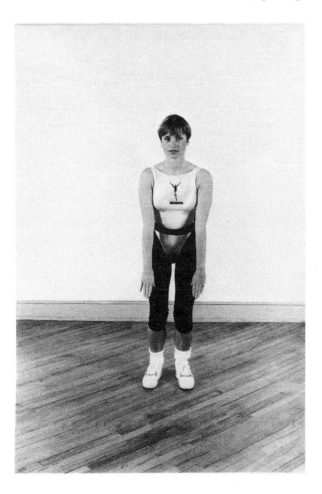

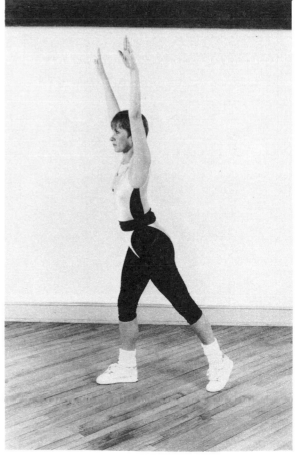

3 LEVEL BLOCK **A**

Repeat

EXERCISE 5

Side to Side Jumps with Arm Swings (p. 120)
4

4

Repeat

EXERCISE 6

Knee Lifts with Arm Pulls (p. 121)
4

4

EXERCISE 7

Spotty Dogs

10

10

• Stand with feet together, jump and split-land with the right foot forward, the left foot back, and with left arm forward, the right arm back, then repeat to land with the left foot forward and the right foot back, changing the arms (1 count)

• Do this 10 times

Do this sequence of exercises five times in order to make a routine lasting 7½ minutes. The first time you perform the sequence, take it easy so as to allow your body time to adjust; work hard for the middle three repeats then use the last time to cool down gently. To get your breath back fully you may need to walk around the room. If you wish you may repeat the sequence more than five times.

Now go to Level 3 cool-down opposite.

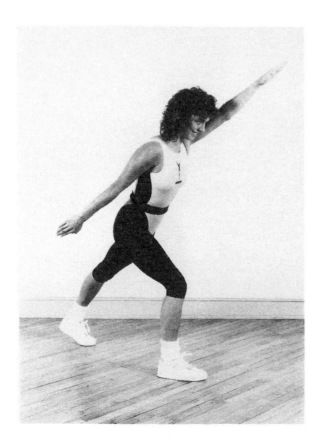

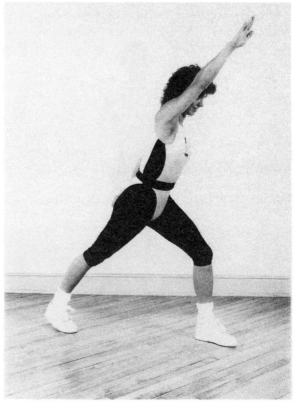

COOL-DOWN

Again, for these exercises you need something comfortable and cushioning to work on. Breathe out as you go into the stretch and concentrate on trying to relax the muscles being stretched. Never bounce or jerk in your stretches; take extra care, as some of these exercises are quite advanced.

The Level 3 cool-down includes a wide variety of short stretches. If you feel you have time, hold these stretches for a little longer as in Level 2.

1½
minutes

EXERCISE 1

Straddle Stretch

PURPOSE: TO STRETCH THE MUSCLES ALONG THE INSIDE AND BACK OF THE THIGH (ADDUCTORS AND HAMSTRINGS)

 8

• Sit on the floor with legs extended as wide apart as is comfortable, and place your hands on the floor in front of your groin

• Keeping the back straight, bend forwards from the hips, and walk your hands forwards until you feel a stretch in the groin and hamstrings

• Hold for 8 counts then release

□ *Keep your knees facing the ceiling*

□ *Ease forwards gently*

□ *Do not expect to get very far down*

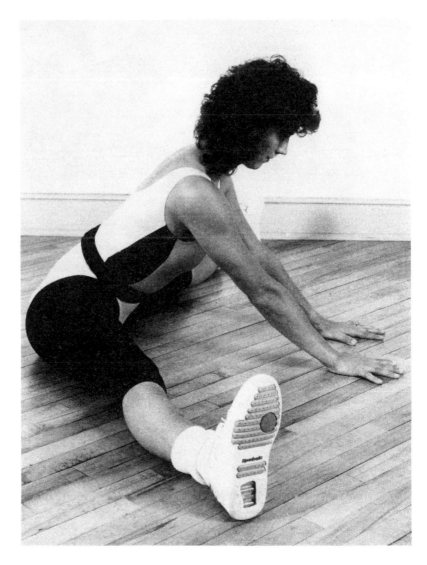

123

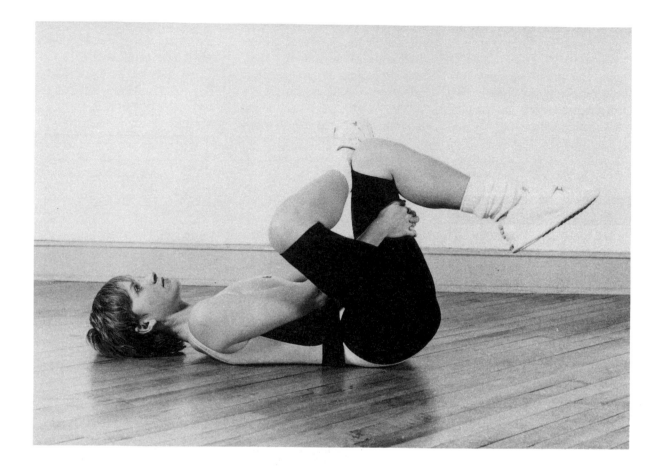

EXERCISE 2

Buttock Stretch

R + L

PURPOSE: TO STRETCH
THE MUSCLES OF THE
BUTTOCKS (GLUTEALS)

16

- Lie on your back and bending the left knee, place the left foot flat on the floor

- Place the right ankle on the left knee and push the right knee away

- Hold the left thigh with both hands and pull it towards you (the legs should then be over your body, with the left foot off the floor)

- Hold for 8 counts then repeat for the left leg

□ *Feel the stretch in the right buttock*

□ *If this is too hard, try keeping the left foot flat on the ground and the right foot over the knee, and sit up (with hands on the floor behind your body), gently easing your body towards the thighs*

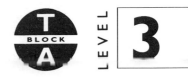

EXERCISE 3

Sitting Shoulder Stretch

PURPOSE: TO STRETCH
THE MUSCLES AROUND
THE SHOULDERS
(DELTOIDS)

8

- Sitting on the floor with bent knees and both feet flat, place your hands flat on the floor behind you with fingers pointing away from your body (see p. 105)

- Bend the elbows slightly and slide your bottom away from your hands until you feel a stretch in the front of your shoulders

- Hold for 8 counts

> □ *Keep the elbows bent*
>
> □ *Place your hands close together*

EXERCISE 4

Lying Stomach Stretch

PURPOSE: TO STRETCH
THE STOMACH MUSCLES
(ABDOMINALS) AND TO
MOBILISE THE SPINE

4

- Lie on your front and place your hands flat on the floor in front of your head, with arms slightly bent (see p. 59)

- Gently lift the head and shoulders off the floor by pushing on your hands and straightening your arms. Keeping your hips on the floor, walk your hands back towards you until you feel a stretch down your stomach

- Hold for 4 counts, keeping your hips on the floor

> □ *Look ahead and keep your hip bones on the floor*
>
> □ *If your back aches, lower your shoulders further or leave this exercise out*
>
> □ *Think of lengthening your spine*

EXERCISE 5

Front-Lying Quad Stretch

R + L

PURPOSE: TO STRETCH
THE MUSCLES AT THE
FRONT OF THE THIGH
(QUADRICEPS)

8

- On your stomach, bring the right heel in towards the buttocks (see p. 93)

- Gently reach for the right ankle with the right hand and pull the heel in further until a stretch is felt in front of thigh

- Hold for 4 counts

- Repeat on the left

> □ *Keep chin, shoulders and hips on the floor*
>
> □ *You might like to stretch both legs simultaneously*

3 LEVEL

T BLOCK A

EXERCISE 6

Kneeling Shoulder Stretch

PURPOSE: TO STRETCH
THE MUSCLES AROUND
THE SHOULDERS

4

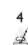

• Kneeling, sit back on your heels then lean forwards so that the chest rests on the thighs (see p. 92)

• Extend the arms forwards and place your hands on the floor in front of you, thumbs close together

• Keeping the chest low, slide your hands and hips forwards, raising your buttocks up off your heels until your hips are directly above your knees

• Push your chest towards the floor and hold for 4 counts

> □ *Feel the stretch around your shoulders*
>
> □ *Keep your stomach muscles tight to prevent the back from arching*
>
> □ *Look down at the floor*

EXERCISE 7

Kneeling Hip and Buttock Stretch

R + L

PURPOSE: TO STRETCH
THE HIP FLEXORS AND
THE MUSCLES OF THE
BUTTOCKS (GLUTEALS).
IMPORTANT FOR
POSTURE

16

• Kneel on your right knee and place your left heel out in front, with the left leg fully extended

• Bend forwards over the left thigh, bending the left knee, and place your hands on the floor on either side of your left leg

---

• Transfer your weight forwards so that the hips are midway between the feet

• Lower the hips towards the floor so as to feel a stretch in the front of the hip

• Hold for 8 counts then repeat for the right leg

> □ *Keep the front foot slightly ahead of the front knee*
>
> □ *To increase the stretch, slide the front foot further ahead and tilt the pelvis*
>
> □ *If your knee hurts with the weight on it, straighten that leg*

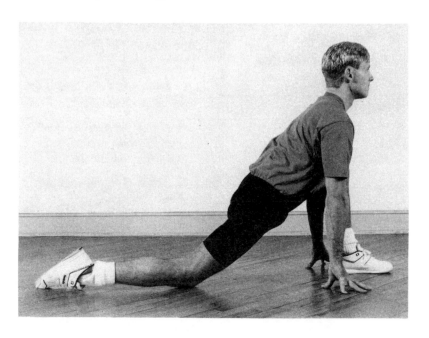

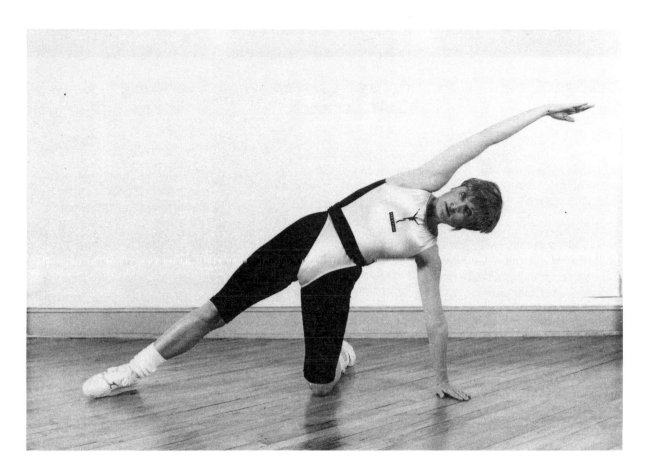

EXERCISE 8

Kneeling Side Stretch

L + R

PURPOSE: TO STRETCH
THE MUSCLES IN THE
SIDE OF THE BODY AND
THE ARMS

8

- Kneel on the right knee and place the left leg straight out to the left side, toes pointed and touching the floor

- Place the right hand flat on the floor, about 18 inches to the right of the right knee

- With your weight balanced between the left foot, right knee and right hand, lift the hips so that they are directly above the right knee

- Curve the left arm over your head to the right to stretch the side of the body

- Hold for 4 counts then repeat on the other side

> ☐ *Keep shoulders, chest, hips and thighs facing front*
>
> ☐ *Keep your hips over the supporting knee and your shoulders over the supporting hand*
>
> ☐ *If this is uncomfortable, do the Standing Side Stretch on p. 104*

3

L E V E L

T BLOCK **A**

EXERCISE 9

Bridge Calf Stretch
R + L

PURPOSE: TO STRETCH THE MUSCLE ALONG THE BACK OF THE LOWER LEG (GASTROCNEMIUS)

 8

- Position yourself with hands and feet on the floor shoulder-width apart and hips in the air, looking at the floor between your hands (see p. 114)

- With the left leg slightly bent and the right leg straight, press the right heel into the floor so as to feel a stretch in the calf

- Hold for 4 counts then repeat on the left

> □ *Push the heel down hard, point the toes forwards and keep the stretched leg straight*
>
> □ *Adjust the distance between hands and feet to increase the stretch; the closer together the harder the stretch*

EXERCISE 10

Bridge Lower Calf Stretch
R + L

PURPOSE: TO STRETCH THE MUSCLE ALONG THE BACK OF THE LOWER LEG (SOLEUS) AND THE BACK OF THE ANKLE (ACHILLES TENDON)

 8

- Assume the same position as for the Bridge Calf Stretch (see p. 115) but bring the feet in slightly closer to the hands

- Bend both legs slightly and press the heel of the right leg into the floor

- Hold for 4 counts then repeat on the left

> □ *Feel the stretch lower down the calf*
>
> □ *Transfer your weight back over the heel to increase the stretch*

EXERCISE 11

Standing Triceps Stretch
L + R

PURPOSE: TO STRETCH THE MUSCLE ALONG THE BACK OF THE UPPER ARM (TRICEPS)

 8

- Stand with good posture and knees slightly bent, curve the left arm behind the head and place the fingers on the upper back between the shoulder blades (see p. 70)

- Using the right hand, assist the stretch by gently pulling the left elbow across behind the head

- Hold for 8 counts then repeat on the other side

> □ *Feel the stretch down the back of the upper arm*

Chapter Five

THE Y PLAN AND LIFESTYLE

'Lifestyle' is one of today's buzz words. The media are full of suggestions about the kind of lifestyle we should be leading and how we could improve it. Put at its bluntest, many commercials suggest that to be wholly acceptable we should all be slim and beautiful, wear chic clothes, drive a fashionable car, pursue a glamorous career, possess tasteful luxury items and relax in the company of similarly fulfilled people.

These images, so relentlessly promoted by the media and by society itself, are not ones that many of us actually conform to, even if we may aspire to them, and often, if we allow ourselves to be pressured into believing that we're not living up to expectations, we suffer from a sense of inadequacy, from confused ideas about what we should be and what we should want. As a result, our self-image suffers too, with an inevitable knock-on effect that further diminishes our lifestyle.

Self-image is related to:

- How we look
- How we feel
- How we cope with day-to-day problems

These three factors are influenced by three aspects of life with which the Y Plan is directly concerned:

- How much we exercise
- What and how much we eat
- Our ability to relax and feel in control

As we have said before, aerobic exercise stimulates the release of endorphins and other chemicals which both improve your state of mind and alleviate physical and emotional tension. The Y Plan really does help you to cope with the stress and anxiety which affect everybody in everyday life.

When Anna joined a Y class she had very little confidence and was about 20 pounds overweight. She hardly ever went out because she had so few friends; she was even having difficulty holding down a job. Within two months of starting the Y Plan, Anna had reduced her weight, without drastic dieting, and therefore she has seen that she has the ability to control her own lifestyle by improving her appearance, her health and her self-image. That success has given her the confidence to be more relaxed with people and now she is a member of a squash club. She also has a regular job – not her first choice, but one she is prepared to stick with until something better comes along. Above all, Anna's family and friends can all see a difference in both her shape and her outlook. She is happier in herself, people are happier to be in her company and, thanks to the Y Plan, she is in control of her life.

Most people will have smaller-scale problems, whether they concern body shape, fitness and energy or feeling relaxed and confident with their lives.

Healthy eating habits, with a balanced, nutritious diet, mean that in combination with regular exercise, you will be able to improve your body shape and feel fitter.

A well-fed body (as opposed to an over-fed body!) will make you feel good and more able to cope with day-to-day demands. It will prevent you feeling tired and you may be less likely to suffer from colds or illness.

Remember, though, that permanent changes don't come in days (whatever some diets claim!). But over weeks and months you will see the difference that sensible eating and sensible exercise make on your life. Make sure you eat the recommended amounts of protein, carbohydrate, fats and fibre each day. Avoid more than a low amount of alcohol and avoid using too many saturated fats. Try to reduce over a period of time the amount of sugar and salt you consume.

COPING WITH STRESS

Stress is often called the twentieth-century disease but it has always been with us under different names. These days we regard stress as a necessary evil of modern living, but stress is not negative – without it, we would not enjoy some of the high points in life. The anticipation before a date, the tension before an important match, the organisation before a party – all these situations produce stress, but provided you can control it and not the other way round you will feel stimulated, not worn down.

Those situations have an obvious positive aspect. However, sitting in a train that is late, being stuck in traffic, working to a tight deadline, coping with financial restraints and relationship problems are much harder to manage or control.

Stress is now recognised as a medical problem and as a significant factor in causing coronary/heart disease, high blood pressure, high blood fats and high cholesterol counts. Dr Peter Nixon of Charing Cross Hospital in London has found, too, that patients are often unwilling to admit to stress problems because they feel they are a form of social failure.

Common signs of stress are increased tiredness, irritability and inability to cope. Rather than prescribing drugs, doctors are now advising activities such as fishing and painting, meditation and exercise as methods of relieving stress.

At Y classes we see many people who appear busy, successful, coping and happy. They may come to us for an apparently simple reason, like the desire to work off a spare tyre, but they stay because regular exercise is so helpful in stress management.

John worked in advertising and because of his long, exhausting day was becoming very inactive. He joined the Y to go swimming once a week, but the exercise made him feel so good that he took up the Y Plan exercise programme. He soon realised that his regular 12-minute Y Plan blocks were something into which he could channel a lot of the tension and frustration caused by high-level negotiations: the physical activity diverted his mind from his problems and simply made him feel better.

HOW TO TEST FOR STRESS SYMPTOMS

To get an idea of the level of stress you may be feeling, you can from time to time ask yourself the following questions and check your rating. Tick one of the boxes for each question then add up your score, counting 3 for every 'Often', 2 for each 'Sometimes', 1 for a 'Rarely' answer and 0 for 'Never'.

Taking a stress scale of 0–75:

Between 0 and 25, you suffer little stress and in any case cope well with it.

Between 25 and 50, you are experiencing quite a significant degree of stress and should consider how you can improve matters.

Between 50 and 75, you are extremely stressed and should seriously consider what lifestyle changes might alleviate this tension.

Of course each person can tolerate different levels of stress, and situations can vary in your life, so the best person to assess your score is always you: don't ask someone else to judge for you. If your score and the way you feel indicate to you that the stress in your life is greater than it should be, the Y Plan Stress Management programme is for you.

HOW TO MANAGE STRESS

The idea is simple and effective. If you follow these basic steps in recognising and avoiding stressful situations, you will find that coping with whatever levels of stress you meet in your particular situation will become much easier.

●1 Learn to recognise signs of stress, such as tiredness and irritability, or others of the points mentioned on p.163.

●2 Listen to your friends and family, because they may be aware of your stress before you are.

●3 Share problems with those around you.

●4 Learn to say no, if saying yes is going to cause an unacceptable level of stress. Saying yes in that situation will mean that you won't give your best.

●5 Be organised. For example, get up 15 minutes earlier if that will mean you don't have to rush or panic.

●6 Allow time for leisure. Develop one or more interests outside work or the demands of home life. Even a long bath or window shopping will take you out of overdrive.

●7 However busy you are, make time for those around you at work and at home.

●8 Remember that no one, not even yourself, is indispen-

	OFTEN	SOMETIMES	RARELY	NEVER
HEALTH				
How often do you:				
● Feel run down or tired?				
● Have difficulty in sleeping?				
● Have stomach complaints?				
● Have back and body pains?				
● Have headaches/migraines?				
● Feel a tightness in the shoulders/jaw?				
WORK				
How often do you:				
● Have frustrated/bad relations with colleagues?				
● Feel vulnerable to criticism?				
● Have a sense of failure?				
● Feel indecisive/overwhelmed by job demands?				
● Feel a lack of enthusiasm for your job?				
● Feel you need more holidays?				
PERSONAL				
How often do you:				
● Feel a lack of enthusiasm and confidence?				
● Feel impatience with the family, flatmates or friends?				
● Become irritated by small things?				
● Feel pressure from people around you?				
● Feel guilt about work-time distracting from family and social life?				
● Feel concerned/anxious about the future?				
● Have feelings of panic?				
● Feel bad temper/loss of sense of humour?				
● Grip a steering wheel tightly?				
● Push back hard into an armchair?				
● Find it hard to relax?				
● Feel easily tearful?				
● Take alcohol or drugs?				
● Feel life is going out of control?				

sable. Things will go on without you.

●9 Go away on breaks and holidays for a change of scene and activity, for the stimulation of experiencing different things in new places.

On a lighter note, two pieces of advice from an eminent American cardiologist:

a. Don't sweat over the small stuff.
b. It's all small stuff.

RELAXATION ROUTINE

Relaxation is a very simple, positive and effective therapy for combating stress. The Y Plan relaxation routine is easily learned and can fit unobtrusively into your life.

Allow yourself the time to learn *how* to relax. Once you have mastered the skill, you can use it at will. The ability to relax really is something you can *learn*; it requires conscious effort to allow physical tension to drain from your muscles, and mental tension to drain from your mind. A great many people say they find it hard to relax, not realising that it is a habit which can be explained and then practised.

The Y Plan approach to relaxation is non-technical. Although it looks like a lot of words, the routine is simplicity itself and easy to memorise:

●1 Find a room where you will be free from interruption for a short time.

●2 Take up a comfortable position where your limbs and body are well supported – in an armchair or on a sofa or the floor.

●3 Close your eyes and stay still for two minutes. Not still to the point of discomfort, of course – an itch can be scratched!

●4 While your eyes are closed, concentrate your mind on each part of your body in turn. As you think of each part, visualise the tension draining out of it and into the chair, sofa or floor.

●5 Start with your shoulders and neck: think about where they are, what they feel like. Can they drop a little? Imagine them sinking into your support.

●6 Now your arms. Let them sink into your support. Register all parts of your arms touching the surface. Think heavy.

●7 Feel your fingers gently touching what is beneath them. Think about their position in relation to each other.

●8 Move down through your back and your bottom. Feel yourself sink deep into your support. Think about precisely which parts of you are touching the surface.

●9 Take your thoughts all the way down your legs to your feet in the same way, letting out all the tension as you become aware of them.

●10 Work your thoughts slowly through all the parts of your body once more, thinking about making them heavy and relaxed and about your entire being sinking into your support.

●11 Next, concentrate on your breathing, the rise and fall of your chest with each breath.

●12 Finally, carefully stretch your arms above your head and inhale deeply. Get up very slowly to avoid feeling dizzy.

When you start your Y Plan fitness programme, try to make time at least once a day for this relaxation routine, especially after exercising, when the muscles are warm. As you become used to doing it you will feel the benefits and soon you will be able to employ the technique in everyday situations, whether or not you close your eyes while you do so – before or after stressful meetings, in traffic jams and as a method of going to sleep.

The Y Plan is a programme for a better lifestyle – a better lifestyle for you. Because it has no strict diet and no single set of exercises, because it doesn't dictate how you should live your life but gives you plans and options, it can be tailor-made for every individual.

By following the Y Plan fitness programme at a level that suits you, you will improve your body shape and fitness. The Y Plan stress management and relaxation routine can reinforce all these benefits and in a few short weeks you will begin to appreciate a change for the better.

The Y Plan is for you, to make you look and feel your best – better than you ever thought possible.

Appendices

Your body is like a machine, with heart, lungs, muscles, bone and blood working together like the pistons, circuits, nuts, bolts and oil of a complex engine. Just as an engine needs regular servicing and adjusting, so the body needs to be properly maintained. Exercise and nutrition provide this. Like machines, each body needs varying kinds of maintenance, so exercise and diet have to be tailored to our individual workings.

The Y Plan deals with three main areas of physical fitness: muscular, aerobic and motor.

MUSCULAR FITNESS

What is muscular fitness? It may seem that if you can get through the day comfortably your muscles must be fit enough already. But there are three aspects to muscular fitness. They affect not only how your muscles work but also how you look. They are: strength, endurance and suppleness. Muscles need to be strong to allow you to perform your activities in an easy and comfortable manner, as well as to give you good posture. If your muscles tire quickly they will often be unable to respond when much more sustained effort is needed. All the muscle-toning blocks of exercise help with this.

If the muscles are too tight, they can restrict your movement: the stretching exercises in the Y Plan will improve your flexibility.

TONING Muscles and fat surround our skeleton; these three are the major factors determining body shape. Exercise that concentrates on repeatedly working specific muscles will strengthen them and improve their shape, consequently improving the shape of your whole body. The process is known as toning.

Exercise is designed to make the specific muscles work harder than normal by repetition of one particular movement. You can feel this yourself by standing tall and rising right up on to your toes twenty times or until you feel your calf muscles ache. This sets up a series of changes in the specific muscles, including improved fuel and blood supply to all parts of them, thereby increasing their capacity to work. Over a period of weeks they become stronger and firmer, giving the body better, more defined shape. If you do not work the muscles for a while – that is, if you neglect your exercise habit – this firmness will vanish and the muscles will become flabby.

It is a myth that unexercised muscle will turn to fat, however. Unexercised muscles do lose their tone but fat is a distinct substance produced by your body as a result of over-eating. It is stored around our vital organs and all over the body under the skin.

You may find the toning exercises less tiring than the aerobic ones in terms of making you breathe hard and making your heart race, but toning exercises are effective when the last couple of repetitions cause the muscles to ache. Either may cause some soreness when you first begin. Remember what you are doing and why.

To understand a little better how your muscles work, imagine two pieces of wood joined at one end by a hinge, and joined in the middle by a length of elastic. The pieces of wood represent bones, the hinge is the joint and the elastic is

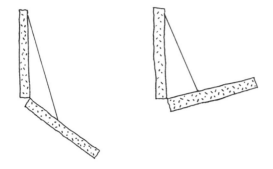

muscle. When the hinge is open the elastic lengthens and when it is closed the elastic is short. Now imagine your arm bent, with the elbow as the hinge and the muscle of the front of the upper arm (biceps) as the elastic. When you straighten your arm the biceps lengthens; to bend your arm you tighten the biceps and it may even result in a little bulge! To complicate matters, there is also another set of muscles on the other side of every joint, so as one muscle contracts, the other lengthens and vice versa.

There are over 650 muscles in the body. The Y Plan selects the most important of these and concentrates on improving them for your needs with the most effective and safe combination of exercises.

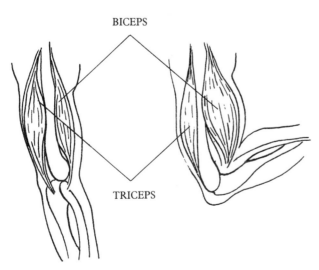

BICEPS

TRICEPS

POSTURE Your body posture is largely determined by the way your muscles support and hold up your skeleton.

Take a good look at yourself in the mirror in your normal standing position.

● Does your chin poke forwards?

● Do your shoulders pull forwards so as to round the top of your back?

● Does your stomach stick out?

● By the end of the day does your body sag?

Round shoulders, a bent neck and jutting head are some of the most common problems among people who don't exercise regularly, along with weak stomach muscles and backache.

Some occupations seem to encourage poor posture. People who spend long periods sitting at a desk or over a typewriter tend to have slouching problems, especially if they don't trouble to see that desks and chairs are at the right height for them.

Working out with the Y Plan will result in improved posture. Your clothes will hang better and you will be able to move more freely and easily. Again, it's a case of feeling better and looking better. Good posture allows you to breathe more easily and reduces strain on the joints and spine. Good posture is fundamental to your fitness and your figure and with the Y Plan it's really quite simple to improve.

Try to remember always to stretch up from the waist and to pull your shoulders back and down. The Y Plan exercises will encourage this as a natural stance and will also strengthen your stomach muscles. These do the vital job of protecting the organs in the abdomen and also of protecting your back. The spine has natural curves that act as shock absorbers, but bad posture (incorrect pelvic tilt) can over-stress these curves by allowing the stomach to stick out and to pull the lower back forwards.

When you improve your posture you reduce the risk of lower backache or injury, and make your stomach muscles firmer and flatter.

When you exercise, always check that:

• You stand with feet shoulder-width apart (unless described otherwise) and with your toes pointing very slightly out on the diagonal (not too much, or you may damage your knees)

• Your stomach muscles are pulled in and your pelvis is correctly tilted (see p. 31)

• Your knees are over your feet

• Your hips are over your knees

• Your shoulders are over your hips

• Your shoulders are pulled back and down but kept relaxed

• You don't exaggerate movements

• You don't force your knees backwards

Do exercise through the full range of movement described in the exercise. There is no benefit in doing things too quickly if it means you don't do them correctly.

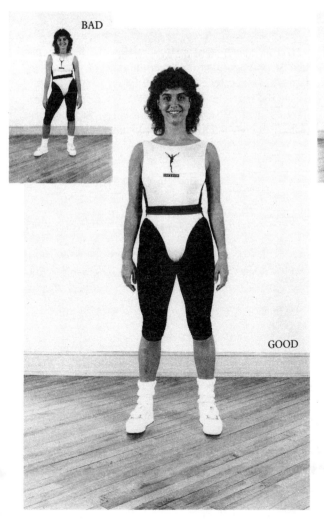

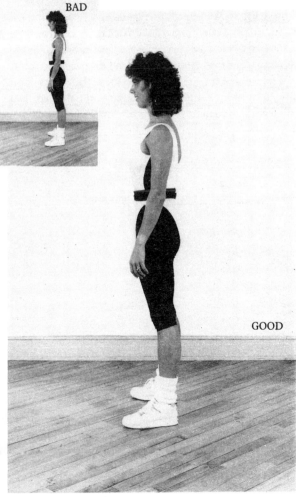

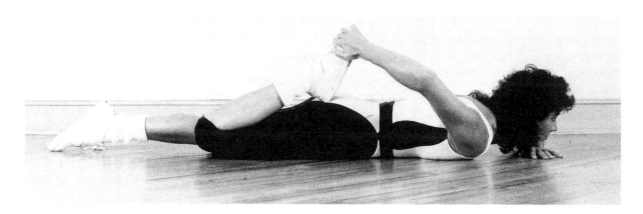

SUPPLENESS   What exactly is suppleness? Does it mean being able to do the splits, to tie your legs round your neck or to touch your toes? Suppleness, or flexibility, simply refers to the range of movement round any particular joint. There are certain ranges of movement that every joint should be able to show and once these are achieved, you can feel that the joint is adequately supple.

For instance, when you lie on your stomach you should be able to touch your bottom with your heels. This exercise relies on the muscles at the front of your thighs stretching adequately. When you lie on your back with one leg straight, you should be able to get the other leg up in the air at 90°. To do this the hamstrings, the muscles at the back of your thighs, have to be sufficiently supple.

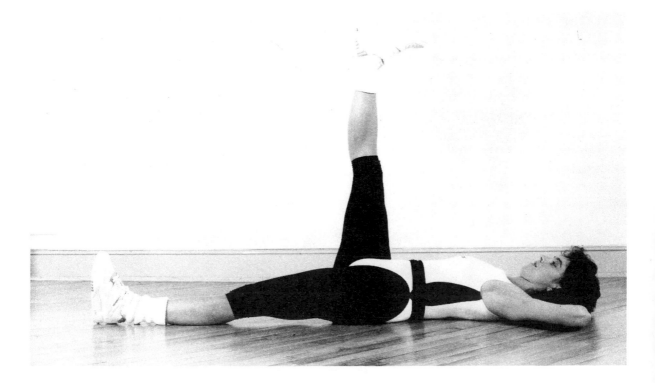

Suppleness is a much neglected component of fitness but when it is improved by the Y Plan exercises you'll find that movement in general will become easier, that your posture will get better and – perhaps less obviously – that you will reduce the risk of all sorts of injury. Exercises for suppleness are based on stretching, which you will also find relaxing. Stretching should always be incorporated in warm-up exercises and as part of the cool-down session after the exercise blocks.

The body has a protective mechanism which shortens muscles and guards against them being overstretched or stretched too quickly. The art is to move slowly and gently, reassuring the muscle that it is safe to stretch. Exercise programmes which include stretching exercises in bouncy, jerky movements can lead to many problems, leaving you feeling stiff and sore the next day at the very least. The Y Plan follows proven, effective and safe stretching methods which allow your muscles to relax gently, thereby gradually improving your suppleness.

AEROBIC FITNESS

Aerobic fitness is another very important component of physical fitness. It is really the basis of healthy living since it relates to the way in which your body is able to cope with various types of everyday activity: walking uphill and running for a bus depend on the state of your heart, general circulation and lungs, all of which benefit from aerobic exercise.

THE HEART   The heart is actually a muscle and like any other muscle it needs to be exercised and it can be strengthened.

Publicity campaigns are constantly urging us to look after our hearts. Why? Because the heart is a pump, and when the pump stops working the whole machine stops working. Heart disease is the No. 1 cause of premature death, so strengthening your heart is just plain common-sense. A strong heart pumps more blood with each beat and so does not need to pump so many times. This means your heart works more effectively in normal circumstances and therefore copes better during exercise.

In recent scientific studies, lack of activity was found to be just as major a factor in coronary heart disease as other well-known dangers like high blood pressure, high cholesterol levels and smoking. The experts conclude that taking exercise which is vigorous, regular and effective can reduce the risk of suffering a heart attack by as much as half.

People who have already suffered a heart attack can also benefit from exercise. A slow, safe, progressive exercise programme can provide positive steps towards recovery and a normal active life.

But make sure that you take your doctor's advice before starting any exercise programme, if you have a heart problem.

GENERAL CIRCULATION   In order to work, your muscles need fuel (foodstuffs and oxygen) in order to release energy. This fuel is transported to them in the blood via the circulatory system which consists of your blood vessels and your heart together. The better this whole system works the more stairs you are able to climb, for instance, and other activities like brisk walking and playing sport also become easier.

If the heart is a pump, then the blood vessels are the pipes connecting the pump to the muscles. Regular exercise keeps the pipes in good condition – it prevents clogging and helps to reduce high blood pressure.

THE LUNGS   The lungs consist of millions of tiny air sacs, which if opened and spread out would cover half a tennis court. They are constantly at work, extracting oxygen from the air and transferring it into the blood. Any damage or deterioration of the lungs will restrict this process.

Smoking is an obvious hazard, as it interferes with the lungs' cleaning system: soot particles in the tobacco smoke, together with the tar, narrow the tiny air tubes and reduce the lungs' function. Smokers become significantly more breathless and also cough readily on the air they do take in as it comes into contact with their obstructed airways, and this is one of the reasons why we are constantly being advised not to smoke.

AEROBIC EXERCISE   The basic aim of Y Plan aerobic exercise is to use some of the body's large muscle groups, like the legs, in order to train the cardiovascular system (the heart, lungs and circulation). These muscle groups require large amounts of oxygen to function properly and so the cardiovascular system has to work harder than usual while you exercise.

If during your exercise you do feel slightly puffed but are still able to hold a conversation, then you're taking it at

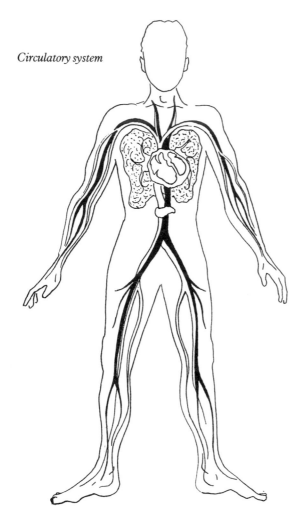

Circulatory system

do not take so long to recover from them. As you become aware of that, remember to notice how much more easily you manage your daily activities.

As well as all the benefits to your heart, lungs and circulation, aerobic exercise can make a big contribution to working away unwanted inches. Another of the effects of sustained aerobic exercise is to encourage your body to burn up fat more quickly and so slim you down all over. It will not work off fat in just one part of your body (or 'spot-reduce') and it won't work miracles in days – no exercise can do either, whatever may be claimed – but as you make exercise a habit you'll find enjoyment in both your increased mobility and your improved body shape.

MOTOR FITNESS

Motor fitness covers a number of aspects of movement: co-ordination, balance, rhythm and speed. Motor fitness is the way your muscles respond to the tasks your mind is asking them to perform and all the Y Plan exercises give you practice in improving your performance.

Have you ever been dancing and trodden on your partner's toes an embarrassing number of times? 'Oh, I can't dance, I'm totally unco-ordinated' is the kind of response we hear often when we suggest that people come to an aerobic class and exercise to music. But moving to music is a skill, and all skills have to be learned. It isn't simply the case that you're born with them or you're not. Almost all the four aspects of motor fitness can be taught and all of them can be improved.

Think how many skills you have acquired in your life – walking, running, feeding yourself, playing sport, using a typewriter, a computer, a knitting machine, a screw-driver. . . .

Everyone learns skills at different rates and some skills suit some people more than others. When we choose our leisure activities we tend to follow the areas which we find easiest, or most satisfying, but that doesn't mean we can't learn the ones we find harder. Top gymnasts, dancers and sports players make their skills look effortless, but think how much training has gone into the process.

Your own Y Plan programme will be balanced to suit your particular needs. It will develop the skills you currently lack and complement the ones you already possess.

the right pace for you. You should definitely not be gasping for breath or experiencing any chest pain. If you do feel such a pain we strongly recommend that you consult a doctor.

Aerobic exercise is all about sustaining a pace for a reasonable time. If you feel like stopping almost as soon as you have started, then you have started too fast, so make sure that you begin slowly enough to give your body time to adjust to the extra activity.

Over a period of weeks, your body will respond to training, and positive changes will occur to the cardio-vascular system. Also your heart will become stronger and will pump more blood out with each beat. All this enables your muscles to work better. You will also notice that you begin to cope more easily with the exercises and that you

FITNESS TEST
Record

Test No.	1	2	3	4	5	6	7	8	9	11	11	12	13	14
TIMED PRESS-UPS														
SIT AND REACH														
TIMED CURL-UPS														
TIMED STEP-UPS														

WEIGHT/BODY MEASUREMENT
Record

Date														
WEIGHT														
UPPER ARM														
BUST/ CHEST														
WAIST														
HIPS														
TOP OF THIGH														
CALF														

L E V E L 1 L E V E L

Week / Date	BLOCK	ASSESS	1	2	3	4	5	6	7	8	9	10	11	12	13	14	15
MON																	
TUES																	
WED																	
THURS																	
FRI																	
SAT																	
SUN																	

L E V E L 2 L E V E L

Week / Date	BLOCK	TRANSITION	1	2	3	4	5	6	7	8	9	10	11	12	13	14
MON																
TUES																
WED																
THURS																
FRI																
SAT																
SUN																

			L E V E L **3** L E V E L													
Week	BLOCK	TRANSITION	1	2	3	4	5	6	7	8	9	10	11	12	13	14
Date																
MON																
TUES																
WED																
THURS																
FRI																
SAT																
SUN																

Cue Card Level 1

Warm-up

1 **SHOULDER CIRCLES** (2 FWD 2 BWD) 16 CTS
2 **ANKLE CIRCLES** (4R + 4L) 8 CTS
3 **KNEE BENDS/ARM CIRCLES** (8) 16 CTS
4 **MARCHES** (16) 16 CTS
5 **HIP CIRCLES** (4R + 4L) 16 CTS
6 **REACHES** (8) 16 CTS
3 **KNEE BENDS/ARM CIRCLES** (8) 16 CTS
4 **MARCHES** (16) 16 CTS

Cool-down

1 **KNEELING SHOULDER** 16 CTS
2 **LYING STOMACH** (2) 16 CTS
3 **SIDE-LYING QUAD** (L + R) 32 CTS
4 **SITTING GROIN** 32 CTS
5 **LYING HAMSTRING** (L + R) 32 CTS
6 **STANDING CALF** (L + R) 16 CTS
7 **STANDING LOWER CALF** (L + R) 16 CTS
8 **STANDING TRICEPS** (L + R) 16 CTS

Warm-up stretch

1 **STANDING TRICEPS** (L + R) 16 CTS
2 **STANDING SHOULDERS** (2) 8 CTS
3 **STANDING CHEST** (2) 8 CTS
4 **STANDING QUAD** (L + R) 16 CTS

Toning exercises

1 **PELVIC TILTS** (6) 24 CTS
2a **CURL-UPS** (8) 32 CTS
2b **REVERSE CURL-UPS** (8) 32 CTS
3a **FRONT LEG RAISES** (8L + 8R) 16 CTS
3b **STANDING FRONT LEG RAISES** (8L + 8R) 16 CTS
4a **REAR LEG RAISES** (8L + 8R) 16 CTS
4b **STANDING REAR LEG RAISES** (8L + 8R) 16 CTS
5a **BOX PRESS-UPS** (8) 16 CTS
5b **STANDING PRESS-UPS** (8) 16 CTS
6 **BUTTOCK SQUEEZES** (8) 16 CTS

Warm-up stretch

1 **STANDING QUAD** (L + R) 16 CTS
2 **STANDING CALF** (L + R) 16 CTS
3 **STANDING LOWER CALF** (L + R) 16 CTS
4 **STANDING SHOULDERS** (2) 8 CTS
5 **STANDING CHEST** (2) 8 CTS

Aerobic exercises

1 **STEP TAP/WITH ARMS** (8 + 8) 32 CTS
2 **WALKS** (4 FWD + 4 BWD/4L + 4R) 32 CTS
3 **TWISTS AND MARCHES** (8 + 8) × 2 32 CTS
4 **SQUAT + REACH** (12) 24 CTS

Cue Card Level 2

Warm-up

1 **HEEL/TOE + ARM EXTENSIONS** (8L + 8R) 16 CTS
2 **SIDE BENDS** (4R + 4L) 16 CTS
3 **SQUAT + REACH** (8) 16 CTS
4 **ARM CIRCLES** (4) 8 CTS
5 **WALKS** (4) 16 CTS
6 **HIP CIRCLES** (4R + 4L) 16 CTS
3 **SQUAT + REACH** (8) 16 CTS
5 **WALKS** (4) 16 CTS

Cool-down

1 **KNEELING SHOULDER** 8 CTS
2 **FRONT-LYING QUAD** (R + L) 32 CTS
3 **LYING STOMACH** (2) 16 CTS
4 **SITTING HAMSTRING** (L + R) 48 CTS
5 **SITTING GROIN** 16 CTS
6 **STANDING SIDE** (L + R) 16 CTS
7 **STANDING CALF** (L + R) 16 CTS
8 **STANDING LOWER CALF** (L + R) 16 CTS
9 **STANDING CHEST** (2) 12 CTS

Warm-up stretch

1 **STANDING TRICEPS** (L + R) 16 CTS
2 **SITTING HAMSTRING** (L + R) 16 CTS
3 **STANDING QUAD** (L + R) 16 CTS
4 **STANDING SHOULDER** (2) 8 CTS
5 **STANDING CHEST** (2) 8 CTS

Toning exercises

1 **STANDING SIDE-LEG RAISES** (6R × 2) 32 CTS
2 **FORWARD SQUATS** (4L) 16 CTS
3 **STANDING LEG-CURLS** (8L) 16 CTS
1 **STANDING SIDE-LEG RAISES** (6L × 2) 32 CTS
2 **FORWARD SQUATS** (4R) 16 CTS
3 **STANDING LEG-CURLS** (8R) 16 CTS
2 **FORWARD SQUATS** (4R + 4L) 32 CTS
4 **STOMACH TWISTS** (10R) 40 CTS
5 **BUTTOCK + LEG SQUEEZES** (12) 24 CTS
6 **PROGRESSIVE PRESS-UPS** (2 × 8) 32 CTS
4 **STOMACH TWISTS** (10L) 40 CTS
5 **BUTTOCK + LEG SQUEEZES** (12) 24 CTS
6 **PROGRESSIVE PRESS-UPS** (2 × 8) 32 CTS
7 **CURL-UPS** (5) 10 CTS

Warm-up stretch

1 **STANDING QUAD** (L + R) 16 CTS
2 **STANDING SHOULDERS** (2) 8 CTS
3 **STANDING CALF** (L + R) 8 CTS
4 **STANDING LOWER CALF** (L + R) 16 CTS
5 **STANDING LUNGE** (L + R) 16 CTS

Aerobic exercises

1 **SQUAT SIDE-STEPS + ARM PULLS** (4 + 4) 32 CTS
2 **KNEE-LIFTS + ARMS EXTENSIONS** (4R + 4L) 16 CTS
3 **DIGS + SKIP BACK** (8) 32 CTS
4 **SQUAT + SWINGS** (16) 16 CTS
5 **TWISTS** (8) 8 CTS
6 **WALKS/BEND + REACH** (4) 16 CTS

Cue Card Level 3

Warm-up
1 **STEP TAP + ARMS** (16) 16 CTS
2 **KNEE LIFT + ARM EXTENSIONS** (4R + 4L) × 2 16 CTS
3 **LEG TAP OUT + ARM SWINGS** (4R + 4L) × 2 16 CTS
4 **WAIST TWISTS** (8) 16 CTS
5 **ANKLE CIRCLES** (4R + 4L) 8 CTS
6 **DOUBLE ARM CIRCLES** (8) 16 CTS
2 **KNEE LIFT + ARM EXTENSIONS** (4R + 4L) × 2 16 CTS
3 **LEG TAP OUT + ARM SWINGS** (4R + 4L) × 2 16 CTS

Cool-down
1 **STRADDLE** 8 CTS
2 **BUTTOCK** (R + L) 16 CTS
3 **SITTING SHOULDER** 8 CTS
4 **LYING STOMACH** 8 CTS
5 **FRONT-LYING QUAD** (R + L) 8 CTS
6 **KNEELING SHOULDER** 8 CTS
7 **KNEELING HIP + BUTTOCK** (R + L) 16 CTS
8 **KNEELING SIDE** (L + R) 8 CTS
9 **BRIDGE CALF** (R + L) 8 CTS
10 **BRIDGE LOWER CALF** (R + L) 8 CTS
11 **STANDING TRICEPS** (L + R) 8 CTS

Warm-up stretch
1 **REAR BEND ARM SHOULDER** (R + L) 16 CTS
2 **STANDING TRICEPS** (L + R) 16 CTS
3 **STANDING HAMSTRING** (R + L) 16 CTS
4 **STANDING SIDE** (R + L) 8 CTS
5 **SITTING SHOULDER** 8 CTS

Toning exercises
1 **LEG RAISES** (16R + 16L) 64 CTS
2 **INTERMEDIATE PRESS-UPS** (12 + 16) 64 CTS
3 **SIDE LEG RAISES** (16L) 32 CTS
4 **TWISTING CURL-UPS + LEG EXTENSIONS** (16L) 32 CTS
3 **SIDE LEG RAISES** (16L) 32 CTS
4 **TWISTING CURL-UPS + LEG EXTENSIONS** (16R) 32 CTS
5 **SIDE LEG RAISES** (16R) 32 CTS
5 **CURL-UPS + LEG** (8R + 8L) 32 CTS
3 **SIDE LEG RAISES** (16R) 32 CTS
6 **CURL-UPS** (16) 32 CTS
7 **DIPS + SQUEEZES** (8S + 8F) × 2 64 CTS

Warm-up stretch
1 **STANDING LUNGE** (R + L) 16 CTS
2 **STANDING HAMSTRING** (R + L) 16 CTS
3 **STANDING SIDE** (R + L) 8 CTS
4 **STANDING QUAD** (L + R) 8 CTS
5 **BRIDGE CALF** (R + L) 8 CTS
5 **BRIDGE LOWER CALF** (R + L) 8 CTS

Aerobic exercises
1 **MARCHES + ARM PUSHES** (1 + 1) × 2 16 CTS
2 **JOG + CLAP** (8) 8 CTS
3 **SQUAT + REACH** (4) 8 CTS
2 **JOG + CLAP** (8) 8 CTS
3 **SQUAT + REACH** (4) 8 CTS
4 **JUMPING KNEE LIFTS + ARM PULLS + SKI SWINGS** (1 + 1) × 4 16 CTS
5 **SIDE TO SIDE JUMPS + ARM SWINGS** (4) 4 CTS
6 **KNEE LIFTS + ARM PULLS** (4) 4 CTS
5 **SIDE TO SIDE JUMPS + ARM SWINGS** (4) 4 CTS
6 **KNEE LIFTS + ARM PULLS** (4) 4 CTS
7 **SPOTTY DOGS** (10) 10 CTS